To Ann

Best wishes

Kittie & Tom

(Kittie Dalton who wrote this book was a patient and a friend of ours. She published many books and gave wonderful parties in her rooms in Harley St London to celebrate the latest publication)

A. J. F.

Premenstrual Syndrome goes to Court

Katharina Dalton FRCGP

Peter Andrew Publishing Company Limited

First edition 1990

Published by
PETER ANDREW PUBLISHING COMPANY LIMITED

ISBN 0 946796 42 4

Typeset in Great Britain by
Steven Graphics,
Droitwich, Worcestershire, England

Printed and bound in Great Britain by
Billings & Sons Limited, Worcester, England

Contents

Preface

'Of making books there is no end; and much study is a weariness of the flesh'.

Ecclesiastes 12:12.

Likewise, it can be said that of the many media presentations and books about the popular misconception of premenstrual syndrome, there is no end and to try to elicit the truth from them would indeed be a weariness of the flesh. However, this is not just another book on premenstrual syndrome, it is a serious study of the legal consequences of the unwitting and unwilling patterns of behaviour among sufferers of premenstrual syndrome and postnatal depression sufferers, which may bring her into transgressions of the law.

Every day the media gives examples of the legal consequences associated with premenstrual syndrome or postnatal depression. It is an area of misunderstanding and confusion. It is hoped that this book will lead to a greater understanding of the problem among the many people, who come into contact with it, either professionally at work, in their family or in their social circle.

The only real names used are those which have had full media publicity and for which there are law reports available to be studied. No confidences have been divulged and the many references of those whose real names appear have been taken from press reports.

I wish to thank all those in the legal, medical and allied professions, who have helped in this publication, and the many who have assisted in obtaining evidence which could be used in court. Special thanks again go to my severest critics, especially Drs. Michael and Maureen Dalton; to Mrs. Wendy Holton for her secretarial skills and the organisation of my appointment schedule to allow me to attend court, and thanks to the next generation who worked so hard on the Index, also Mrs. Anita Dalton, who put the original manuscript on disc. As with all my other publications I have had the unstinted help of my husband, Rev. Tom Dalton, who with his familiarity with dictionaries and word finders has put the right word in the right place, and tried to ensure that my wildly scattered punctuation marks came to rest where they should.

It is my sincerest wish that the enlightenment this book brings will help thousands of women worldwide.

London, 1990 Katharina Dalton

Foreword

As the reader of this book will find out, the concept of using a medical disease or, in some cases, a set of symptoms as mitigation for crimes committed is not a twentieth century legal phenomenon. Women have been acquitted of crimes, because of peculiar circumstances surrounding their behavior at the time of menstruation, in the last century as well as this one. However, it is only in recent years that we have begun to understand more clearly the relationship of certain behavior patterns to the recurrent cyclical episodes of menstruation. Much of the medical profession's present knowledge of this relationship stems from the pioneering work of the author of this volume, Dr. Katharina Dalton. It was she, in my opinion, more than anyone else who brought the myriad of symptoms associated with menstruation into a logical and coherent focus, and it is her collected works that form the basis of our present interest in Premenstrual Syndrome.

Readers who are familiar with Dr. Dalton and her 'style' will immediately recognize the following: 1) The text is 'pure Kittie Dalton', with generous helpings from her husband, Tom; and 2) the importance of establishing a correct diagnosis, which point Dr. Dalton has stressed over and over in her written as well as in her oral presentations.

Dr. Dalton's style is factual, but the reading is easy. Science and case histories are interwoven most effectively. Perhaps no other practitioner has seen as many women who suffered from severe Premenstrual Syndrome as Dr. Dalton, and she has called on some of the most interesting case vignettes to assist in enlightening the reader.

With regard to making an accurate and correct diagnosis anyone who has taken the trouble to read Dr. Dalton's other work will remember this has always been the cornerstone upon which she rests her advocacy of progesterone therapy . The problem as I see it is that many people who quibble with the use of progesterone have not taken the time to understand the rationale underlying its suggested use. It should be clear that if the patient doesn't have the disease, it is unrealistic to think that the therapy will work.

Dr. Dalton is to be commended for stressing that she is not advocating the use of Premenstrual Syndrome as a wholesale 'cop-out' for any woman who has been charged with an offence. She has laid down strict criteria for the approach to an offender in whom there may be even the slightest possibilty that Premenstrual Syndrome was a mitigating factor, she points out that the majority of individuals who raise the spectre of Premenstrual Syndrome as a defence can not substantiate it. For these women and their lawyers, Dr. Dalton provides no great comfort. On the other hand, for the few women who suffer from the severe form of the disease and in whom it can be documented, this book should be a welcome ray of hope. It should also serve as a beacon for all those concerned with rehabilitation of the sick as well as the criminal. Dr. Dalton points out near the conclusion of this volume that the use of Premenstrual Syndrome as a defence implies that therapy is necessary and demands that the court supervise this therapy as any part of its judicial process.

Dr. Dalton's comments about the Food and Drug Administration's stance on progesterone as it relates to Premenstrual Syndrome are well taken. Clearly the FDA has a mandated responsibility to insure that the American public receives drugs that are safe as well as efficacious . Although there is no question about the safety of progesterone, it would appear that the FDA is not convinced about its efficaciousness. The difficulties of assessing the need for clinical trials, the selection of appropriate patients, requirements for blinding, controls, stratification, and cross-overs are beyond the scope of this volume and certainly outside the area of expertise of most practicing physicians.

As a practicing Obstetrician/Gynecologist it is within my purview to mention to the readers of this volume that I have met Dr. Dalton on several occasions, heard her lecture, and have attended her offices in London. I continue to be amazed at the breadth and scope of her knowledge and experience with this disease. Letters and 'phone calls from grateful patients and doctors come from all over the world. It is highly unlikely that this would be the case unless both the patients and the physicians who referred them were satisfied with the advice they received.

As Dr. Dalton has pointed out, we are just beginning to scratch the surface of understanding Premenstrual Syndrome. It is now clear that not everyone suffers from it throughout their entire lives, that the disease can wax and wane with time, that certain events aggravate it or precipitate an exacerbation and that the patients respond differently to therapy. It is also clear that progesterone by itself is not the only medication for all women. Perhaps it will be said in the future that Dr. Katharina Dalton's greatest contribution was to bring Premenstrual Syndrome to the attention of her colleagues, to champion the plight of its victims, to suggest a form of therapy that works for many many patients, and then to sit back with a sense of pride knowing that other workers will also make their own contributions.

If one looks at Dr. Dalton's clinical practice, her writings, her teaching, and now this volume, one can justifiably say, 'Well done, Kittie'.

Professor Louis Keith, M.D.,
Head of Section of undergraduate
Education & Medicine,
North Western Student Affairs,
North Western University Medical School,
Chicago.

1

Introduction

The criminal aspect of premenstrual syndrome (PMS) was brought to the attention of the British public in 1980 when two women charged with murder and one charged with arson were set free on probation with a treatment order.

Murder, arson and false emergency calls harassing the police, what common factors link these three cases?

1. They were committed by young women.
2. Their Counsels had successfully pleaded premenstrual syndrome as a mitigating factor in their crime.
3. At the time they committed their offence none of them was aware that they suffered from premenstrual syndrome.

In each case it was the father, not the woman herself, who had noticed the cyclic repetition of the uncontrollable behaviour of his daughter each month. All three women were seen initially by the author whilst they were in custody in the prison cell and they agreed only reluctantly to the preliminary examination. All three women suffered from premenstrual syndrome and were restored to normality as law abiding citizens by progesterone treatment (Dalton 1980). The definition of premenstrual syndrome is ***the recurrence of symptoms before menstruation with absence of symptoms after menstruation***.

These three women represent a minute proportion of those women whose mood swings prior to menstruation are so violent that for a short time each month they are no longer responsible for their actions. They represent the extreme end of the spectrum of premenstrual syndrome, which ranges from normality, through mild symptoms which may include forgetfulness, and the making of sarcastic remarks or a quick rebuff, to exceptionally severe psychological changes including confusion, violence, delusions and hallucinations over which they have no control.

Nevertheless those few women who, for an hour or a day or

two each month, do lose control of themselves need help and help is available. These rare individuals must not be confused with the remaining 99.9% of women who have other premenstrual symptoms, nor with the lucky majority who have no symptoms whatsoever related to the menstrual cycle. It is axiomatic that not all sufferers from premenstrual syndrome are criminals and that not all women criminals suffer from premenstrual syndrome.

The acceptance of premenstrual syndrome as a factor, which may lead to diminished responsibility or mitigation, at law, places a particular responsibility upon the medical and legal professions (and also on society) to ensure that justice is carried out and that treatment is provided to those suffering from extremely severe premenstrual syndrome. At the same time, it is the responsibility of both professions to make sure that there is no abuse of the law thereby allowing malingerers to escape the consequences of their actions. This book has been written to assist physicians and lawyers in discharging their responsibilities. It is not a handbook to help guilty people to escape justice, neither does it intend to provide excuses for those who break the law. Above all it makes no pretence at teaching law to the legal profession or medicine to the medical profession. However, in order to alert professionals who are likely to be involved in the defence and prosecution, or observation and treatment of sufferers from severe premenstrual syndrome, it is crucial to understand the precise definition and methods of diagnosis of this common condition which can bring women, unwittingly and unwillingly, into committing 'a legal wrong that can be followed by criminal proceedings, which may result in punishment'. Premenstrual syndrome is a disease which responds admirably to the correct prophylactic treatment with progesterone, restoring the woman to a normal and useful life as a law abiding member of the community.

The acceptance of premenstrual syndrome as a mitigating factor in the causation of anti-social and/or criminal behaviour has led many people to fear that the floodgates have been opened to an endless succession of pleas, which claim premenstrual syndrome in mitigation, thereby trivialising the plea.

Even when premenstrual syndrome has been correctly diagnosed, that fact alone does not provide grounds for mitigation. It still needs to be established that the premenstrual symptoms are of the type and severity to account for the alleged offence. Every woman who believes she is suffering from premenstrual syndrome, of such severity that there is a serious risk of harming herself or others or is in danger of damaging property, has a duty to seek, accept and follow through any treatment schedule prescribed by a competent physician. Nevertheless, all too often the sufferer is unaware of the precipitating causes of her episodic and strange behaviour and so rationalises her temper tantrums onto someone else, usually her nearest and dearest. It will then be for others, namely the husband, family members, workmates, social workers, health visitors and doctors to make the connection between the recurrent symptoms and menstruation. The responsibility then becomes theirs to persuade the sufferer to seek treatment, a task which may need to be postponed until the postmenstruum when normality has been regained.

The recognition of premenstrual syndrome as a medical disease, with the appreciation of the extreme severity of some of its symptoms, is not only of benefit to women.

In 1979, a 29 year old man was accused at Winchester Assizes of murdering his fiancee one evening in a car. The fiancee was described as a polecat who, at certain times each month, would become aggressive and attack him. On the night in question, she started to hit him and, to protect himself, he put his hands around her neck and held her until she became quiet.

In fact she became quite quiet and died of strangulation, but the man was freed on the grounds that he was defending himself against the violent effect of her premenstrual syndrome. As to the justice of this judgement, I leave the readers to decide when they have finished reading the book.

❑ Reference

Dalton K. (1980). *Lancet 2;* 1070-1071.

2

The Law and Premenstrual Syndrome

Premenstrual syndrome is accepted in Great Britain as a cause for diminished responsibility in a charge of murder and as a mitigating factor in other criminal and civil crimes (*R. v Craddock*: *R. v English*: *R. v Owen*). The occurrence of premenstrual syndrome has not yet been tested in this manner in the courts of the United States, although in Calgary, Canada, it has been accepted as a mitigating factor in a charge of shoplifting.

The acceptance of diminished responsibility allows a charge of manslaughter to replace that of murder, but it clearly is a guilty plea to the offence. A guilty plea of murder carries a mandatory life sentence in Great Britain. However, if a person is guilty of manslaughter then it is up to the judge to determine the punishment, which can vary from imprisonment to probation. Even if the defendant is released on probation she still has a criminal record. It should be apparent that the distinction is based on diminished responsibility and not absence of responsibility. In diminished responsibility and mitigation the degree of diminution may vary from 5 to 100%. At present the premenstrual syndrome is not accepted as a legal defence in Britain; if it were then the defendant would be left without the stigma of a criminal record. Probation has shown itself to be a valuable device to ensure that treatment is continued, which may be necessary for the protection of the public. A method of removing the stigma of a criminal record is to apply for a Queen's pardon.

It needs to be recognised that it is only an insignificant minority of women whose extreme sensitivity to the hormonal changes of menstruation causes their behaviour to become potentially dangerous. However, just because menstruation is for most women an ongoing but comparatively unmomentous part of their daily life, those few who do suffer must not be forgotten. Premenstrual syndrome has been called a non-disease, an imaginary disease, or a syndrome of social expectation. Every woman menstruates and most women have learned to live with it, and there are those who feel that all women must learn to control their rages, temper tantrums and pains for fear that the recognition of premenstrual syndrome may cause men to regard them as endocrinological cripples. It has even been suggested that it is better that a few premenstrual syndrome sufferers should unjustly spend the best part of their lives in a prison cell, rather than criminals be able to successfully use a false plea and go free. However, this is not an either/or situation. There is a middle ground and this book is aimed at helping both the prosecution and the defence counsel to ensure that equal justice is available to all women.

Owen, Craddock and English were different cases showing the way premenstrual syndrome can produce bizarre effects on a woman's life. Their cases will be discussed in the relevant chapters of this book as it discloses the evidence that was required, how it was obtained and the treatment given leading to the judges' decision of a probation order.

In the earlier case of *R. v Owen* premenstrual syndrome was accepted in mitigation in a case of arson (Dalton 1980), whereas in *R. v Craddock* and *R. v English* premenstrual syndrome was accepted as diminished responsibility for murder. There are important differences in the cases for whereas Misses Owen and Craddock were unaware that they suffered from premenstrual syndrome, although it was recognised by their fathers, both had suffered since puberty and had a history of recurrent episodes of strange and sometimes criminal behaviour and neither of them had any symptoms of premenstrual bloatedness, weight gain nor headaches. In both instances previous imprisonments did not deter these women from further instances of misbehaviour. In contrast Mrs. English had a long history of premenstrual syndrome but this was her first offence.

In April 1982, an attempt was made by Mr. Keith Evans, the barrister, who defended Craddock, to make premenstrual syndrome a legal defence. Miss Smith previously known as Miss Craddock had, since puberty, committed 45 offences, appeared before court on 28 separate occasions, and attempted suicide more than twenty times. She had been seen by 23 psychiatrists who had all reported to the courts that she had no psychiatric disorder and was fit to attend trial. She had been seen by numerous doctors. She was defended on the grounds that her criminal acts had been irresistible impulses caused by the hormonal imbalance of premenstrual syndrome. An irresistible impulse is a situation in which a person knows what she is doing, knows that she ought not to be doing it but cannot restrain herself from doing it. While acknowledging the hardships suffered by one unable to control her violent impulses due to a disease of the body, the judges at the Court of Appeal in London ruled that protecting society had a higher priority than preventing a women being unfairly branded as a criminal. Thus premenstrual syndrome cannot provide a woman with a defence for crime, but it is a powerful mitigating factor.

The basic principles of criminal law require two elements; *'actus reus'*, the guilty act, and *'mens rea'*, the guilty intent. The *mens rea* must be purposely, knowingly, recklessly or negligently. If *mens rea* is not present at the time of the action the finding is one of 'guilty by reason of insanity'. Because in Britain a plea of insanity, including temporary insanity, requires that the offender remains in corrective protection, e.g. Broadmoor, for Her Majesty's pleasure, an insanity plea is not a defence any sufferer of premenstrual syndrome will lightly choose, although it was considered in the first court appearance of *R. v Owen*, when it was adjourned for further medical advice. In this case however Miss Owen was diagnosed, treated with progesterone and released on one year's probation, (Dalton 1980). Oleck (1952) states that in France the premenstrual syndrome 'fits into the legal criteria of temporary insanity', but there do not appear to be any records of its use as a defence. In the United States the defence of premenstrual syndrome has not yet been tried on a capital charge. The admission of a new scientific principle in law depends on the general acceptance by the particular speciality in which it belongs. The Americans have been slower to accept premenstrual syndrome as an endocrine disease and although the Federal Drug Administration has accepted the safety of progesterone suppositories, no manufacturer has yet shown the efficiency of progesterone suppositories in American clinical trials.

❑ References

Dalton K. (1980). *Lancet 2;* 1070.
Oleck H. L. (1952). *Int. Rec. Med. Gen. Pract. Cli;* 166,492.

3

Characteristics of Crimes and Offenders

Offences committed by women during the premenstruum, when they are suffering from premenstrual syndrome, have three major characteristics; they display spontaneity, are irrational or are associated with violence. All three characteristics are interrelated and have interrelated processes – loss of insight; amnesia; confusion; delusions; and loss of control. Some of these characteristics are inherent in premenstrual syndrome offences such as shoplifting, baby battering, child neglect, road traffic offences, alcoholism, hoax telephone calls, arson, assaults to the person and damage to property. However, even if all the characteristics are present in any one offence, it still requires the sequence of events to conform to the strict requirements of the diagnosis of premenstrual syndrome (Chapter 6).

The characteristics all imply a temporary absence of the essential thought processes required to formulate the necessary intent, which would mean, in legal terms, that there was no *'mens rea'* or guilty intent. The state of mind of an untreated premenstrual syndrome sufferer in her paramenstruum has often been described as being 'out of control', which is exactly why premenstrual syndrome is referred to in America as 'the dyscontrol syndrome'.

All these characteristics are in reality those of premenstrual syndrome, which in itself is not the criminal offence. The offence is the resultant effect of the influence of these characteristics on the individual's behaviour at that particular time of her menstrual cycle. However, premenstrual syndrome crimes also have particular distinctive qualities. These could be listed as:

Recurrent offences
The offence is committed alone
It is not premeditated

There is no apparent motive
There is no attempt to escape detection
The offence is committed when there has been a long interval without food.

Sometimes the action may be a 'cri de coeur', which is fully described in Chapter 10.

❑ Recurrent offences

Characteristically, the same or similar offences will be committed with each menstrual cycle, because it will be the same underlying premenstrual symptom precipitating the irresistible impulse that produces the offence, whether it be confusion, lethargy, depression, or irritability. There may be an interval of one or more cycles intervening without an offence, nevertheless the premenstrual symptoms will still occur, and it should be possible to produce evidence of the occurrence of the premenstrual symptoms and/or the increased alertness after menstruation.

The poison pen letter writer has paranoid thoughts relating to some injustice, real or imaginary. These thoughts come to the surface each premenstruum when she has an uncontrollable impulse to write a letter, usually malicious or offensive. Some months she may post the letter, on other occasions she drops it in the letter box of the recipient herself, and there may be times when she is able to unburden herself to a friend or neighbour so that no action is taken. If she is suffering from premenstrual syndrome the intervals between the letters will be multiples of the length of her usual menstrual cycle, so that if her usual cycle is 30 days the letters may be posted at intervals of 30, 60 or 90 days.

A violent outburst, which entails smashing a shop window, will result in police proceedings, but when the same woman smashes up items in her own home, or even the home of a friend, police proceedings are less likely to be instigated. Again, intervals between offences may be multiples of the length of her usual menstrual cycle.

The depressed childless mother who, in the depths of despair and seeking her heart's desire, illogically buys baby clothes hoping this will hasten the day when she has her own baby, or on another occasion takes items of babyfood for which she has not paid, or even tries to steal a baby, is also acting under an irresistible impulse, for her actions are forced upon her by the same delusional symptoms each cycle.

M. D. was a medical secretary aged 32 years. She was charged with her first shoplifting offence. She had quarrelled with her husband on the way to the shopping centre. Her plea was that it was due to the irritability of premenstrual syndrome and that she couldn't remember what happened after she got out of the car. Her husband gave evidence that although this was her first offence, she had these monthly temper tantrums when her whole personality changes during the premenstruum and she becomes confused. This had only occurred since her recovery from postnatal depression after the birth of her second child, now aged 15 months. Even if she was at home all day she would still get confused doing the housework, like scrubbing the kitchen floor a second time although leaving the beds unmade, or setting the table for a meal and placing the polishing cream and Windolene next to the condiments. It was a recognised joke in her household, but they did not realise that treatment was available. Now under treatment with progesterone she is a different woman and a model housewife. Recurrence of amnesia and confusion had clearly been confirmed by the husband and family, although this was her first offence.

Premenstrual syndrome in the young teenager can be present in a different way.

At a boarding school north of London a fire was discovered in the cloakroom after afternoon school. No one was hurt although there was some damage to the property. The following month a small fire was discovered in the dormitory one evening. It did not prove too difficult to discover the girl responsible, who had been menstruating on both occasions.

❑ Offences are committed alone

Offences due to premenstrual syndrome are committed alone,

never with others. It is no defence for one woman charged with four men in a bank robbery to claim that she was in her premenstruum. Hallucinations, delusions and confusion are very personal symptoms. Even when such symptoms are so compelling that they cause anti-social behaviour, they are still only experienced by that individual.

> In 1981, a 34 year old vagrant and an unemployed man with whom she was living were both charged with the murder of an elderly man in his lodgings. They went prepared to burgle the house, complete with fire lighting equipment so that it would appear to be an accidental fire. She was in her premenstruum at the time and wished to plead diminished responsibility due to premenstrual syndrome.

Although the offence occurred during her premenstruum there was no evidence to support her plea for premenstrual syndrome. In cases such as these it was easy to show that there was no evidence of a cyclical recurrence of offences nor were there any underlying premenstrual symptoms triggering an irresistible impulse.

❑ The offence is not premeditated

The offence is not premeditated, and rarely is there any evidence of planning before the offence. The act usually comes as a surprise to those who were present shortly before the incident.

> Craddock, the barmaid referred to in Chapter 2, who was charged with fatally stabbing another barmaid as she was walking home from work, is an example of this. The defendant and the victim had both received some harsh words from a third barmaid, who slapped the victim in her face and kneed her in the groin and the defendant sprang to her defence. She and the victim then walked off talking together, but only a few yards further up the road the defendant stabbed the victim. The defendant left the scene but was found wandering in a dazed condition in north east London. She was only partly coherent during the hours that followed the incident. What had suddenly caused the defendant to stab the friend she had just been

defending a few minutes earlier in the previous quarrel and assault? Others, who had been with her at the public house that night were amazed at what the defendant had done. The two girls had always been the best of friends. The irresistible impulse occurred during the premenstruum and may have been an auditory hallucination.

❑ The action is without apparent motive

Not only is the offence not premeditated, but it is without apparent motive. The action can only be understood if one has knowledge of the particular delusion that the patient is labouring under at the time of the act. If an internal voice is perpetually ordering a person to do some unusual or antisocial act she may finally obey.

A woman had visited a friend in Southend. On her return to the station to catch a train back to London, she suddenly threw a brick into a shop window for no apparent reason. She could not even remember what type of shop it was nor why she had done it. She started menstruating the next day.

❑ No attempt to escape detection

The normal reaction of a person who has committed a crime is to avoid detection, to run away from the scene, to hide the stolen goods or find a receiver, to arrange a disguise or an alibi. However, if the person who has committed the offence is suffering from premenstrual syndrome, the amnesia, confusion or lack of insight eliminates any appreciation that an offence has been committed or is being committed and there is no compulsion to escape detection. The woman mentioned in the last example, who threw a brick through a shop window, went to a telephone box and called the police, informed them of what she had done and dutifully waited at the telephone box for the police car to take her to a police station. There are many similar examples with arsonists who will raise the alarm, and report the fire they themselves have caused, and wait patiently by the telephone box to be arrested. This action and the previous one may well be a 'cri de coeur'. Chapter 10 is devoted to this subject and covers cries for attention, love and sympathy presenting as acts of attempted suicide, self mutilation, arson and some obvious cases of shoplifting.

❑ Long food gaps before the offence

The offence is usually committed when there has been a long interval without starchy food, the interval may well exceed six to eight hours immediately prior to the offence. The effect of this for a premenstrual syndrome sufferer is fully discussed in Chapter 11, but a brief explanation is that when the blood sugar drops too low spurts of adrenalin occur, causing the blood sugar level to rise. Adrenalin is the hormone of fight, fright and flight, and when adrenalin accumulates it may result in uncontrollable violence, confusion or amnesia. The woman's diet is usually poor, especially devoid of starchy food, and often the pangs of hunger have been kept at bay with prolonged heavy smoking. If this is accompanied by insufficient sleep the effect of the long food gap is intensified. The lack of breakfast is common among shoplifters apprehended at midday or early afternoon, while family violence is more frequent when the husband returns home late at night and the wife has been waiting for a meal together. In *R. v English* the defendant had been on a pub crawl all afternoon and evening consuming non-alcoholic drinks, but she had no food for 9 hours prior to crashing her car into her lover.

❑ Analysis of premenstrual syndrome violence and criminal offenders

In 1983, a survey by the FDA into the safety and efficiency of progesterone prophylaxis for premenstrual syndrome, called for an analysis of 1,095 well diagnosed premenstrual syndrome patients (Dalton 1984), seen personally by the author during that year and successfully treated with progesterone therapy, either currently or during the past 35 years. This revealed that out of 984 women who were under 45 years of age at the time of the first interview, 38 of them had been charged with criminal acts during the premenstruum. A further 68 women had admitted to premenstrual violence; 32 women with premenstrual alcoholic bouts; and 22 were premenstrual psychotics.

Table 3.1 Offences committed by women with premenstrual syndrome (n = 38) (designated as offenders)

Assault to person		20
Arson		7
Damage to property		6
Theft		6
Alcohol		6
Disorderly conduct		4
Beyond parental control		
School truancy	2	
Nymphomania	2	4
Hoax phone calls		3
Drugs		3
Homicide		2

(Some women committed more than one offence)

Table 3.1 shows the variety of crimes with which the 38 women had been charged. Many had offended more than once, and often there were different offences. There was a difference between those who had been charged with assault and the other 68 women who admitted to being violent in the premenstruum in that while 53% of the offenders tended to assault people, 94% of the other violent women damaged property and not persons. However, whereas violence to police, employers, teachers and neighbours may result in a criminal charge, violence to her husband or a child is not necessarily reported (Table 3.2).

Table 3.2 Assault to persons and damage to property by offenders and violent women with premenstrual syndrome

		Offenders	Violent women
n		38	68
		%	%
Assault to	police	11	-
	husband	14	6
	child	16	5
	others	12	-
Total assault to persons		53	11
Damage to property		34	94

(Not all offenders were violent)

The offenders tended to be younger; 53% of them were under 25 years of age at the time of their first consultation compared with 13% of psychotics and 9% of the violent women. The alcoholics were in the older age group; 61% aged between 36 and 45 years at their first consultation (Table 3.3).

Table 3.3 Incidence of age, parasuicide and self-mutilation in PMS

	Offenders	Alcoholics	Violent	Psychosis	PMS Series
n	38	32	68	22	984
	%	%	%	%	%
Under 25 years	53	-	9	13	14
26-35 years	37	39	45	63	47
36-45 years	10	61	46	24	39
Parasuicide	37	25	17	36	6
Self mutilation	13	-	-	-	0.1

(Dalton 1984)

D'Orban and Dalton (1980) noted that the average age of the violent women they studied in prison was also young, averaging 24.6 years with a mean age of menarche at 12.3 years and a range from 9 to 15 years.

In a Japanese study by Endo and colleagues (1978) all seven women with menstrually related periodic psychosis were of a young age, 13-23 years, and they all made a complete recovery within 1-11 years. Only two case histories are given; one aged 19 years had visual hallucinations and delusions of reference with the onset of her first menstruation.

Referring back to the analysis, (Table 3.3), it is interesting to note the high incidence 37% of attempted suicides among the offenders compared with other groups, and that self mutilation (slashing the body, and stabbing) was limited almost totally to the offenders (13%), with only one other woman among the 984 sufferers of premenstrual syndrome (0.1%) having reported a single instance of wrist slashing. Among the self mutilators, recurrence of the injury was the rule rather than the exception, and many had their scars removed at a later date after treatment and full recovery.

Eighteen women offenders under 25 years of age with a criminal record were seen during 1982 (Dalton 1984). The first recorded instance of their anti-social behaviour occurred within an average of eight months after their first menstruation, but it was only after court appearances or imprisonment that the diagnosis was made. On the average this was some five years later (Table 3.4). As a consequence of delayed diagnosis, treatment was started only after five years of misery and suffering. These young women were fortunate that once their hormonal balance was corrected, they could start sorting out their muddled lives.

Table 3.4 Early antisocial behaviour noticed in young premenstrual syndrome offenders (n = 18)

Patient	Age PMS first diagnosed	First Record of antisocial behaviour	Start of abnormal behaviour	Age of Menarche
	Years		Years	Years
JP	16	Expelled from school	14	13
AF	20	Depressed, wouldn't come out of bedroom for one week	11	11
MW	19	Hoax phone call	14	12
JD	14	Violent, beyond parental control	12	11
HT	19	Overdose	13	11
LL	19	Fantasised rape	14	14
HR	18	School truancy	13	12
CB	15	Violent, ripped off dress at second menstruation	11	11
BM	22	Expelled theatre school	13	12
NO	18	Overdose	14	13
JD	24	Overdose	11	11
SE	15	Hit teacher, expelled	13	13
TR	22	Overdose at boarding school	15	14
EM	16	Suspended from school	12	11
JJ	17	Violent, hospitalised at menarche	13	13
AS	17	Expelled from school	11	11
JS	21	Overdose	13	12
SB	17	Violent	14	13

The reason for the tragic delay in recognising these 18 young offenders, who were not diagnosed or treated until they had acquired a criminal record, may relate to the popular image of premenstrual syndrome occurring predominantly in the mid-thirties age group (Figure 3.1). In 1957 Lloyd suggested premenstrual syndrome should be called the 'Mid Thirties Syndrome'.

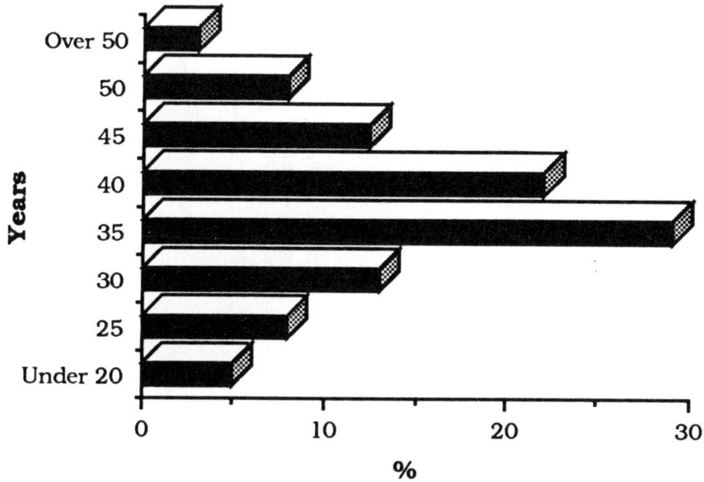

Figure 3.1 Ages at first visit of 1,095 severe premenstrual syndrome patients

In their prison study of 50 violent women, D'Orban and Dalton (1980) pointed out that only two were aware of any possible connection between their menstruation and their aggressive behaviour and that of the 22 women who offended in the paramenstruum less than one quarter had premenstrual symptoms. They emphasised that it is *the cyclically recurrent, observable behavioural changes, of which the woman herself may not be aware, that should be looked for rather than subjective symptoms reported by the patient.* These authors added that some patients may benefit from progesterone or other forms of treatment.

❑ Premenstrual dullness

Premenstrual dullness is another characteristic of premenstrual syndrome which also has a bearing on criminal offences, especially shoplifting. Premenstrual dullness was reported in a study of 1,560 weekly grades of girls at a boarding school. It was found that there was an average drop of 10% in performance during the premenstrual week with a rise of 20% in the postmenstrual week (Dalton 1960) (Figure 3.2).

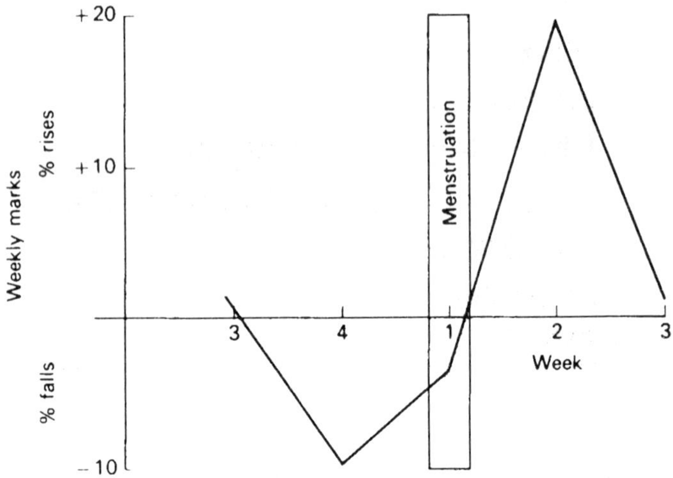

Figure 3.2 Variation in schoolgirls' marks due to menstruation *From Dalton, K. (1960) British Medical Journal 2, 1647-1649.*

This premenstrual fall and postmenstrual rise in academic performance was present equally in all age groups tested from 11 to 17 years. It was equally present among the bright and the dull girls and equally distributed among the consistent and inconsistent performers. It is presumed to result from the lethargy and slow recall some schoolgirls experience in the premenstruum and early menstruation.

Other studies have shown that schoolgirls are more likely to be punished during the paramenstruum (Dalton 1961). This is not to say that the schoolgirls are all well behaved during the rest of the month. It is quite possible that they are naughty during the rest of the cycle but are not caught because they are in their alert phase. If a whole class of pupils are talking as the teacher enters, the alert pupils will immediately stop talking and sit down, while those in their duller phase with slower reaction time will continue talking and be punished. This same principle may well operate in certain criminal events, such as shoplifting, where alertness is vitally important.

❑ References

Dalton K. (1960). *Brit Med J;* **2**, 1425-1426.
Dalton K. (1961). *Brit Med J;* **2**, 1752-1753.
Dalton K. (1984). *Premenstrual Syndrome and Progesterone Therapy* 2nd Ed. William Heinemann Med. Bks Ltd/Year Book Medical Publishers Inc. Chicago.
D'Orban P. J. & Dalton J. (1980). *Psychol Med;* **10**, 353-359.
Endo M., Daiguji M., Asano Y., Yamashita I & Takahoshi S. (1978). *J. Clin. Psychiat;* May 456-466 .
Lloyd T. S. (1963). *Virg. Med. Month* 90, 51.

4

The Normal Menstrual Cycle

When reading through some 24 papers prepared for discussion at a conference held in Philadelphia in September 1984, on the 'Legal and Ethical Implications of Premenstrual Syndrome', it was astounding to realise that most contributors seemed completely unaware of the variations of normal menstruation. Amongst the twenty four eminent speakers were psychiatrists, psychologists, geneticists, philosophers, one physiologist, a sociologist, an attorney, a social worker, a criminologist and two obstetrician/gynaecologists, only these two would have had any daily intimate knowledge of the variations of normal menstruation and the different types of menstrual flow. This basic information is necessary for a full appreciation of premenstrual syndrome and this chapter has been written to fill any gaps in the reader's knowledge.

To most people, menstruation represents the disintegration of the lining of the womb which is flushed out in the menstrual flow. In this enlightened age we are taught that the menstrual cycle normally lasts 28 days and this is the length of cycle for which the contraceptive pill is designed. However this is not normal menstruation for taking the pill has created an artificial cycle. To understand normal menstruation one must start with the brain. At the base of the brain is an area known as the hypothalamus which is where the menstrual controlling centre is situated (see Figure 4.1). The menstrual controlling centre establishes the length of the menstrual cycle for that particular individual and the timing of all the events taking place within that cycle.

From the menstrual controlling centre, stimuli pass to the pituitary gland, situated adjacent to and below the hypothalamus. The pituitary's task is to synthesise numerous hormones which, as chemical messengers, pass to various organs of the body. Two of these hormones pass to the ovaries; they are the follicle stimulating hormone (FSH) and the luteinising hormone (LH) respectively. The FSH stimulates ovarian cells to produce another hormone, oestrogen, which stimulates the maturation of a single minute egg cell, or ovum each month. The oestrogen also passes to the womb (uterus) where it acts by causing growth of the lining of the uterus (endometrium).

As the ovum matures it passes from the centre of the ovary to the surface where a small blister or cyst is formed. When the ovum is mature and the endometrium is ready a sudden spurt of the second pituitary hormone, LH, stimulates the release of the ovum which then passes down the fallopian tube to the uterus, and hopefully is fertilised on its way. Meanwhile the tissue from which the ovum was released is programmed to make a special hormone, progesterone. This hormone helps to make the endometrium ready to receive the fertilised embryo.

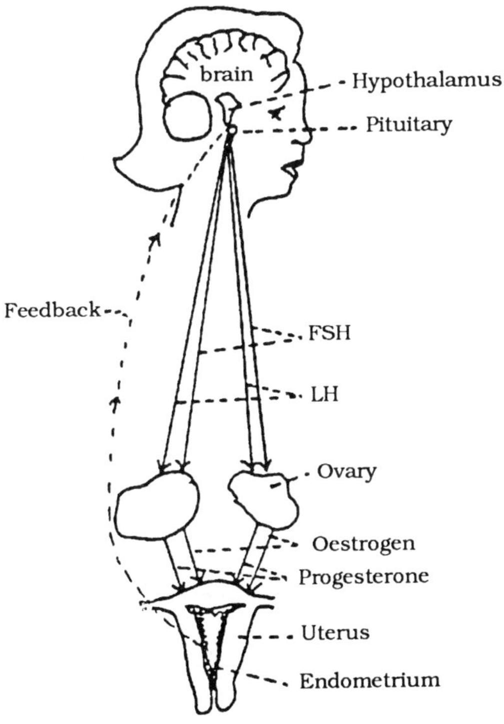

Figure 4.1 Hormonal pathways of normal menstruation

Progesterone also has an important function in regard to sugar metabolism (Chapter 12).

At all stages of the hormonal pathway there exists feedback mechanisms which serve to keep all organs fully informed of hormone levels, causing increases if the level falls or slowing production if a high level is reached.

❑ Menstruation is failed pregnancy

In reality, menstruation is a failed pregnancy. If conception does not occur within the seven days following ovulation, the level of progesterone falls and there is a gradual disintegration of the thickened endometrium (Figure 4.2). It is this disintegration of cells which constitute the menstrual flow.

However, if pregnancy does occur, there is an immediate and rapid rise in the level of progesterone and also the other menstrual hormones, such as FSH, LH and oestrogen, this rise continues throughout the next nine months. Progesterone is initially produced by the ovary. Later this function is taken over by a new, specially formed organ called the *placenta*. The placenta produces vast amounts of progesterone, reaching some 30 to 50 times the level of progesterone found at the peak of the premenstrual luteal phase of the cycle (the 14 days from ovulation to menstruation) in a normal woman who is menstruating. It is not surprising, with these high levels of progesterone during pregnancy, that sufferers from premenstrual

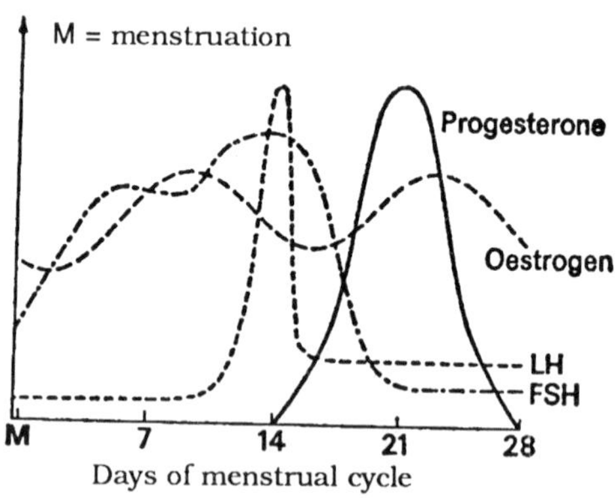

Figure 4.2 Levels of sex hormones in the menstrual cycle.
From Dalton K. (1980) Depression after Childbirth.

syndrome report they are completely free from their symptoms during this nine month period of pregnancy and describe their state of health as the best ever (Figure 4.3).

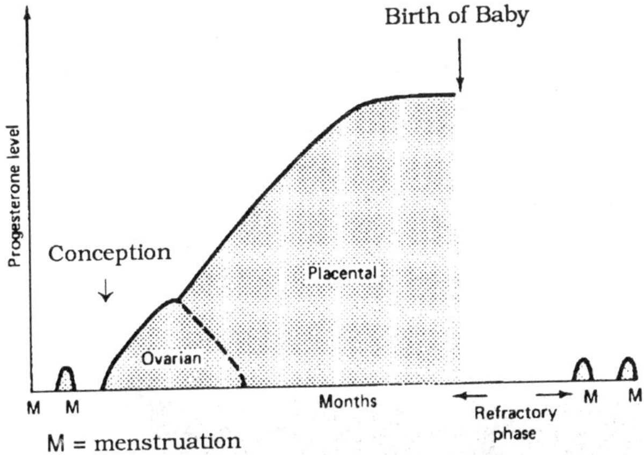

Figure 4.3 Levels of progesterone in the menstrual cycle and pregnancy

Although the discussion presented above is merely a basic outline of a normal menstrual cycle, it must also be appreciated that from the brain to the uterus other processes are taking place to maintain the continuity of this cyclical process. In addition it must be realised that there are other cells in the body which require oestrogen and progesterone for their normal functioning.

❑ Number of menstruations

The number of menstruations a healthy woman can expect during her menstruating life, that is from menarche to menopause, has increased dramatically over the years. One hundred years ago life expectancy was lower, malnutrition was rife, chronic debilitating illnesses were common and women bore larger families. Roger Short, quoted by Pollitt (1977), pointed out that women bearing ten children and breast feeding for the then accepted prolonged intervals could expect an absence of menstruation for 27 of an average potential of 35 menstruating years. In sharp contrast is today's mother of two, who rarely breast feeds for longer than three months and therefore will only have two years freedom from menstruation during the same interval of time (Figure 4.4).

Throughout the childbearing years, normal menstruation is accepted as having variations in length of plus or minus four days cycle by cycle, with an average menstrual cycle lasting between 21 and 36 days. For example a woman with cycle lengths of 32, 30, 34 and 31 days in 4 consecutive cycles would be considered to have normal regularity of menstruation. Thus considerable variations exist both between individuals and within the same individual. Unfortunately, the biology teaching in schools and in common texts assumes a cycle of 28 days, which is the average of all cycles. In fact, in no age group does the precise 28 day cycle occur on more than 16% of occasions,

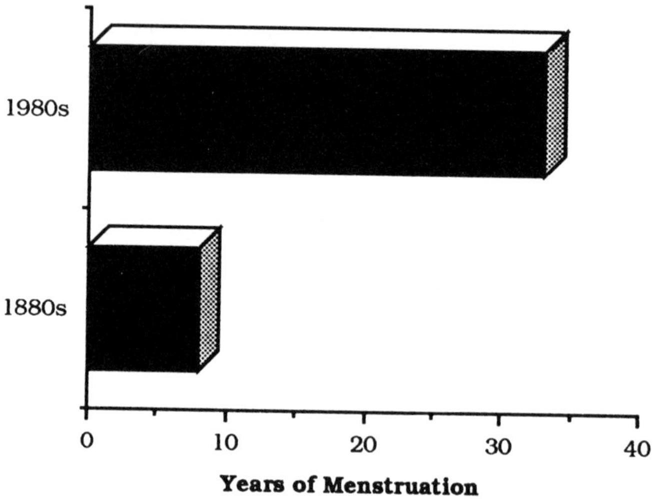

Figure 4.4 Expected years of menstruation in 1880 and 1980

and a degree of irregularity of less than six days occurs in a mere 13% (Wilson & Rennie 1976). Therefore, it must never be assumed that the cycle is 28 days. Too many investigative surveys into the physiological components of menstruation have made this erroneous assumption. Kerr *et al* (1980) did clinical trials on the treatment of premenstrual syndrome and limited their subjects to those with regular cycles of 26 to 30 days, thereby eliminating a large proportion of healthy women with normal menstruation.

The regularity of menstruation increases with age. A mean cycle length of 25 to 31 days was found in slightly more than 60% of 15 to 19 year olds. This increases to 85% in women between 35 to 39 years (Chiazze 1968). As the luteal phase of the cycle (from ovulation to the start of menstruation) remains relatively stable at 14 days, the length of the menstrual cycle is largely determined by the duration of the follicular phase (from the onset of menstruation until ovulation). The length of the follicular phase progressively shortens with increasing chronological age, averaging 14.2 days in the 18 to 24 years group and diminishing to an average of 10.5 days for the 40 to 50 years group (Lenton *et al* 1984).

❑ Menstrual flow

There are also variations in the quantity of menstrual flow day by day during menstruation. Some women experience their heaviest flow on the first and second day, and then the blood loss decreases over the next two to four days. Other equally healthy women have only a very slight loss on the first day or two and then a heavy flow for a few days. There are endless variations of normal. Indeed, in a few women the flow stops entirely for one or two days and then restarts. These variations of normal are important in any consideration of premenstrual syndrome, for there is relief of symptoms with the full menstrual flow, but, in those women who experience only a slight loss for a few days at the beginning of menstruation their symptoms may continue into menstruation. In fact these women are in menstruation chronologically, but in their premenstruum physiologically.

Menstrual blood does not normally clot as it contains no fibrinogen. Although there may be apparent clots in the vagina, these are accumulations of red cells clustered onto a mass of mucoid material. Often these appear as small darkly coloured masses in the vagina and are common if there is a heavy flow. The menstrual flow may appear as bright red, fresh blood, or as dark red, brown or black. These variations reflect the time elapsed since the blood left the endometrium. If the entrance to the uterus (cervix) is wide open, the blood will be bright red, whereas if the opening is narrow and the flow slow in coming down into the vagina, the blood will appear darker.

In a study of 92 women; Chimbira and his colleagues (1984) found that there was no correlation between the woman's subjective assessment of whether her menstrual blood loss was light, medium or heavy, compared with the laboratory measurement of the true blood loss as determined by collecting all sanitary pads and tampons used.

The reader will now begin to appreciate, in view of the variations in length of menstruation, duration of menstrual flow, day of heaviest flow, as well as age and parity, some of the many difficulties encountered in clinical research and therapeutic trials. It is indeed well nigh impossible to accurately match a control subject with the same length of menstruation, duration of flow, day of heaviest flow, age and parity.

❑ Ovulation

Menstruation normally occurs fourteen days after ovulation regardless of cycle length. Given these circumstances ovulation does not necessarily occur exactly at midcycle. The precise timing of ovulation can best be determined by measuring the time of the sudden short-lived rise of LH. A less reliable method is by taking the temperature each morning before getting out of bed, (known as the basal temperature). A sudden drop is followed by a rise at the time of ovulation, but this method is not so reliable. However, ultra sound scans of the ovaries are very accurate.

❑ Menstrual synchrony

Menstrual synchrony occurs when two women have similar menstrual cycles with their menstruations occurring at the same time. This phenomenon commonly occurs among women living together. It is especially liable to occur in prisons, hostels, university campuses and with mothers and daughters. It is most marked among close friends and room mates rather than among random pairs. (McClintock 1971).

❑ Effect of stress

Stress may alter the normal menstrual cycle, but the exact

alterations which occur vary from one individual to another. The effect of stress was demonstrated on 91 boarding school girls who all sat for their 'O' level examinations (English school leaving examinations normally taken at 16 years) during the same days in June. At this school, girls routinely recorded the dates of their menstruations in a book set aside for this purpose, so each girl's normal menstrual pattern was known from menarche onwards. The stress effect of examinations was shown by a sudden increase in the number of girls menstruating during the examination period (Figure 4.5). During May an average of 16 girls menstruated each day; however the number of menstruating girls rose abruptly during examination week, reaching a maximum of 36 girls menstruating on 19th June, the day when the maximum number of examinations were held. Eleven girls had a cycle shortened by four or more days from their norm, 19 girls had a cycle longer than their norm by four or more days and a further eight girls missed menstruation entirely that month. Thus, the stress of examinations caused a significant alteration in the normal length of the menstrual cycle in 42% of candidates (Dalton 1968).

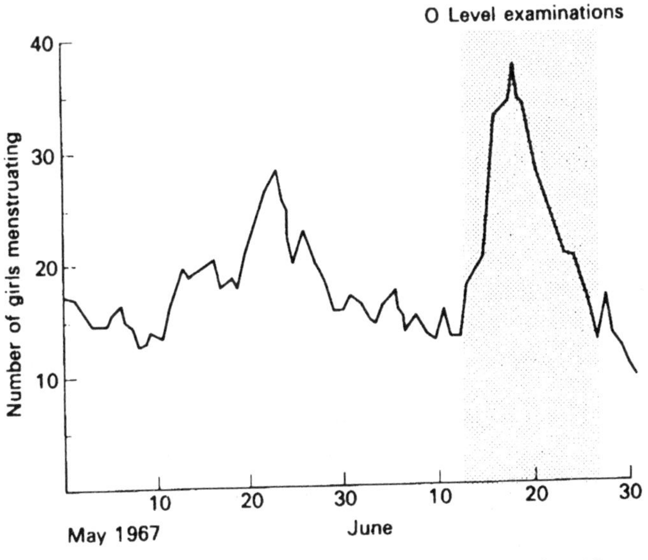

Figure 4.5 Time of menstruation of 91 examination candidates. *From Dalton K. (1968). Lancet; ii: 1386.*

This study of schoolgirls confirmed the well recognised phenomenon that the same stress, in this case examination, can produce different and even opposite effects in different individuals. Furthermore, the result of stress on each woman's menstruation appears to remain the same throughout her menstruating life. Those who experienced absence of menstruation at 16 years are likely to react to stress in later life with missed menstruation or scanty menstruation, whereas those whose cycles were shortened at 16 years are more likely to react with shorter cycles and those who had a heavier loss may have flooding, a condition known as 'weeping womb'.

This varying response to stress is shown in Figure 4.6 and 4.7. It is the menstrual chart of a 43 years mother of two children, who on August 20th moved to a new house half a mile away. Her menstruation was due on the day of her move, instead she missed that menstruation entirely. She resumed her normal pattern in September with menstruation starting on the day that would have been expected had there been no interruption (Dalton 1969).

By coincidence a mother of similar age, also with two children, had to move her home from London to the Sussex coast on August 17th. She became very tense and worried at all the planning involved in the move. The effect of this stress gave her a prolonged menstruation lasting 18 days, but the normal pattern was restored within two months as she settled into her new home (Dalton 1969).

It must be appreciated that the stress of a criminal episode or court appearance can easily upset the normal menstruating rhythm.

❑ Menarche

In Britain the age of the first menstruation, or menarche, covers a wide span, ranging from 10 to 15 years, the average being 13.1 years. The figures for most European countries are similar but, in the United States the figure is around 12.5 years with a range from 9 to 17 years (Bullough 1981). The onset of menstruation is influenced by weight, racial, genetic, dietetic, social and economic factors. There is an earlier average menarcheal age of 12.2 years among those attending special

	Jan.	Feb.	Mar.	Apr.	May	Jun.	Jul.	Aug.	Sep.	Oct.	Nov.	Dec.
1												
2												
3												
4												
5												
6												
7												P
8												P
9											P	P
10											P	P
11										P	P	
12										P	P	
13										P		
14										P		
15												
16									P			
17									P			
18									P			
19									P			
20							P	X				
21							P					
22						P	P					
23						P	P					
24					P	P						
25					P	P						
26					P							
27					P							
28												
29												
30												
31												
Total												

P = period X = moving house

Figure 4.6 Missed menstruation on house-moving day.
From Dalton (1969) 'The Menstrual Cycle' - Penguin Books.

schools for the deaf and blind in Britain, with an even earlier average menarcheal age among those with physical handicaps traceable to early foetal life, like spina bifida and rubella (Dalton & Dalton 1979). The first menstruation usually lasts from three to eight days, which is rather longer than most of the menstruations of the girls' own mothers. Irregularities are common in the first two years of menstruating life. Only about

	Jan.	Feb.	Mar.	Apr.	May	Jun.	Jul.	Aug.	Sep.	Oct.	Nov.	Dec.
1												
2												
3												
4												
5												
6												
7												
8												
9												
10								P				
11								P				
12								P				
13								P	P			
14								P	P			
15								P	P			
16								P	P			
17							P	PX	P			
18							P	P	P			
19							P	P	P		P	
20					P		P	P	P		P	
21					P	P	P	P	P	P	P	P
22					P	P	P	P	P	P	P	P
23					P	P	P	P	P	P	P	P
24						P		P	P	P		P
25								P				
26								P				
27								P				
28								P				
29								P				
30												
31												
Total												

P = period **X** = moving house

Figure 4.7 Prolonged menstruation at the time of house-moving. *From Dalton (1969) 'The Menstrual Cycle' - Penguin Books.*

four menstruations occur in the first year. Even by the age of 16 years, 20% still have cycles which last longer than 40 days, and 33% have menstrual bleeding for at least seven days.

❑ Menopause

The end of menstruation, or menopause, occurs between 45 and 55 years, and is usually preceded by lessening of the menstrual flow and occasionally missed menstruations. At the menopause the ovaries stop their production of oestrogen and progesterone and terminate any feedback from the ovaries to the hypothalamus and pituitary. This causes the pituitary to overact in an effort to stimulate the ovaries back into action, and a marked increase occurs in the blood levels of FSH and LH (Figure 4.8).

The symptoms of the menopause are quite different from premenstrual syndrome. Menopausal symptoms are continuous, whereas premenstrual syndrome symptoms are cyclical with normality in between. Menstruation becomes lighter at the menopause, if heavy loss or flooding occurs it is pathological and requires gynaecological advice. The characteristic symptoms of the menopause include flushes with hot sweats at night; thinning of the skin causing wrinkles and of the vagina causing painful intercourse and frequency of urination; aching joints particularly of the fingers and toes; and stiffness on rising in the morning. The flushes are sensations of heat arising from the waist, passing up to the face and lasting about five minutes, only one or two may occur in a week or there may be up to thirty in one day. Before the flushes there is often a sensation of apprehension and anxiety. In addition psychological symptoms include forgetfulness, confusion and depression, these symptoms may be responsible for criminal acts. The diagnosis of the menopause may be made by measuring the level of the FSH, which is raised while the oestradiol level is reduced.

❑ Pregnancy

When pregnancy occurs there is an immediate rise in all hormones, especially progesterone. Initially the increased progesterone comes from the ovary, but gradually the placenta is formed within the uterus, this produces massive quantities of all hormones, especially progesterone. Initially there may well be an increase in premenstrual symptoms at the time of

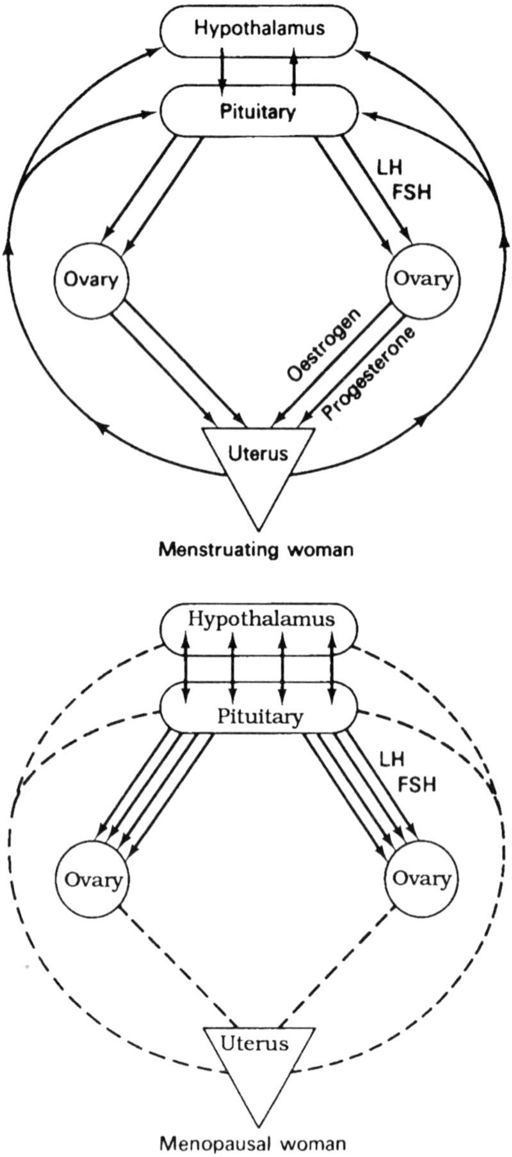

Figure 4.8 Hormonal pathways in menstruating and menopausal women. *From Dalton K. (1984) 'Premenstrual Syndrome and Progesterone Therapy' 2nd Edition.*

the first missed menstruation, but later in pregnancy premenstrual symptoms disappear the woman usually feels her best ever during the second half of pregnancy. However at birth with the delivery of the baby the progesterone-producing placenta also comes away and suddenly within one day the progesterone blood level drops to zero. Those women who cannot adjust to this abrupt loss of hormones may develop postnatal depression.

❑ Postnatal depression

Postnatal depression may be defined as 'the first psychiatric illness occurring within six months of delivery', and it starts at times of hormonal change such as occur at delivery, on stopping breastfeeding, with the first menstruation and on starting the oral contraceptive pill. After childbirth menstruation is usually delayed until breastfeeding has stopped for a couple of weeks. As postnatal depression improves this improvement is initially in the postmenstruum with a return of symptoms after ovulation, then month by month there is a gradual improvement and absence of symptoms in the postmenstruum until it changes into premenstrual syndrome. In 1985 a study was reported in San Francisco of more than 300 women, who had previously suffered from postnatal depression, in whom as many as 84% had subsequently suffered from premenstrual syndrome confirmed by a three months menstrual chart (Dalton 1989).

The Infanticide Act of 1939 states that a mother cannot be found guilty of the murder of her child within twelve months of birth. In practice this means that she is not charged with murder, for if she pleads guilty to that she must have a custodial sentence; instead she may be charged with manslaughter for which she can have a sentence ranging from custodial care to probation or complete freedom. It is important to note that the Act only covers murder of her child and not the murder of another person. If postnatal depression is present the first menstruation can be very traumatic, preceded with severe premenstrual symptoms which may not previously have been present. In practice it is found that criminal acts during postnatal depression occur either within the first two weeks of childbirth or during the premenstruum. Because of the close correlation between premenstrual syndrome and postnatal depression (PND), in the Netherlands, their treatment centres are known as 'PMS/PND Clinics'.

❑ References

Bullough V. L. (1981). *Science;* **213,** 365-366

Chimbira T. H., Anderson A. B. M., & Turnbull A. C. (1984). *Brit. J. of Obst Gynaec.;* **87**, 603-609.

Chiazze L, Brayer F. T., Macisco J. J., Parker M. P., & Diffy B. J. (1968). *Amer J. Med. Ass.;* **203**, 377-380.

Dalton K. (1968). *Lancet 2;* 1386-1388.

Dalton K. (1969). *The Menstrual Cycle*, Penguin Books Ltd., Harmondsworth, England.

Dalton K. (1989). *Depression after Childbirth*, Oxford University Press, 2nd Edition.

Dalton M. E. & Dalton K. (1978). *British Med.J.;* **4**, 475

Kerr H. D., Day J. M., Munday M. M., Brush M. H., Watson M. and Taylor R. W., (1980). *Practitioner;* **224**, 852-855

Lenton E. A., Landgren B. M., Sexton L., & Harper R. (1984). *Brit. J. of Obst Gynaec;* **91**, 681-684

Pollitt J. (1977). *Proc. Roy. Soc. Med.;* **70**, 145-148

Wilson E. W. & Rennie (1976). *The Menstrual Cycle*, Lloyd-Lu, Ke (Medical Books) Ltd., London.

5

Definition of Premenstrual Syndrome

An essential preliminary before premenstrual syndrome can be universally accepted at law is the strict adherence to a precise definition. More than 30 years of research into premenstrual syndrome has produced a clear and precise definition.

'Premenstrual syndrome is the recurrence of symptoms in the premenstruum with complete absence of symptoms in the postmenstruum'.

The essential criteria demanded by this definition are:

1. Cyclical recurrence of symptoms.
2. Their presence in the premenstruum.
3. Their complete absence in the postmenstruum.

Evidence will be required in respect of each of these three points.

The presence of menstruation is a prerequisite. The definition excludes girls whose menstruation has not yet started, those whose menstruation has stopped, whether due to anorexia or taking hormonal contraception, especially the long acting injections, those who are pregnant, have had a hysterectomy and/or removal of their ovaries, and those past the menopause. Women in these groups may have cyclical episodes of bizarre behaviour, even to the extent of having an offence recorded, and they may well respond admirably to progesterone therapy, but technically this is not premenstrual syndrome. It is rather that their symptoms are due to a cyclical hormonal imbalance, and stricter evidence of their symptoms and condition will be required.

❑ Recurrence of symptoms

For general purposes, this means that a recurrence of symptoms must have occurred at the same time in each of the last three consecutive menstrual cycles. This is a minimum requirement. The first question that needs to be answered by any woman claiming that her shoplifting was due to premenstrual syndrome is "What did you shoplift last month?" If her response is a positive one, then you want to know about the previous month or months and try to pinpoint the actual dates. Usually, the shock of that one question, together with an explanation of the definition of premenstrual syndrome, is enough to cause many women to go away and think of some other defence. It is not necessary for the offence to have been the same, nor indeed for an offence to be committed every month, but the underlying premenstrual symptom needs to be the same.

Furthermore the abnormal behaviour will repeat itself while the woman is detained in prison, as occurred in *R. v Craddock*, and *R. v Owen*. Many a woman sentenced for causing grievous bodily harm, arson, hoax telephone calls or shoplifting will repeat the same abnormal behaviour in the next premenstruum, maybe within a few days of her release. This confirms that, *the punishment of a prison sentence is no deterrent for behaviour which is beyond the individual's control.* Premenstrual syndrome sufferers are also the ones who repeatedly tend to lose remission for good behaviour and tend to serve their full sentence.

❑ Limitation of symptoms in the premenstruum

Strictly the term 'premenstruum' refers to the days immediately before the full menstrual flow (page 25). The conventional 28 day cycle can conveniently be divided into seven four-day phases, with each phase having a different level of oestrogen and progesterone (Table 5.1). Most of the studies linking events with the time of the menstrual cycle have used these seven phases.

As already mentioned in Chapter 4, a short or long cycle is a reflection of the length of the follicular phase, and any adjustment is made in the early or late postmenstrual phase.

In medical literature, one may find many other interpretations of the term 'premenstruum', which literally means 'before menstruation'. Asso (1978) reviewed 36 studies on arousal in the premenstrual phase and noted the wide variation covered by the term premenstruum, which included periods of one, two, three, four, and seven days before menstruation; as well as the 'luteal phase'; 'from ovulation to one day premenstrually'; late secretory phase'; and 'one day premenstrually and the first day of menstruation'. However, in premenstrual syndrome, the premenstruum covers the whole of the menstrual phase, from ovulation to menstruation, which can never be more than 14 days. Symptoms of premenstrual syndrome increase in severity from ovulation to menstruation and the most severe symptoms which could be responsible for a criminal event occur in the four days immediately before menstruation. (See paramenstruum page 38).

Table 5.1 Seven four-day phases of the menstrual cycle

Days	*Phase*	*Oestrogen*	*Progesterone*
1-4	Menstruation	Low	Absent
5-8	Early postmenstruum	Rising	Absent
9-12	Late postmenstruum	High	Absent
13-16	Ovulation	Falling	Low
17-20	Early luteal	Rising	Rising
21-24	Late luteal	High	High
25-28	Premenstruum	Falling	Falling

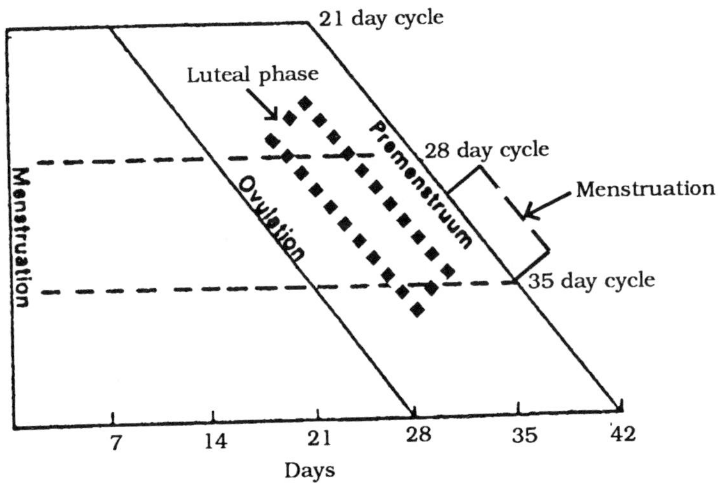

Figure 5.1 Timing of ovulation with different lengths of menstrual cycles

Occasionally an incident occurs in the morning with, menstruation starting later in the day. If further enquiries are not made it may appear that the incident occurred during menstruation.

Symptoms of premenstrual syndrome abate with the onset of the full menstrual flow. In those cases where there is a scanty loss or only slight spotting of blood at the beginning of menstruation, the symptoms should be counted as occurring in the premenstruum as this is physiologically the premenstruum, although chronologically it is menstruation. It is precisely for this reason that the term 'paramenstruum' was introduced (Figure 5.2).

❑ Paramenstruum

Paramenstruum covers the last four days before menstruation and the first four days of menstruation.

These are the days most at risk of those events which are affected by menstruation. Surveys have shown an unduly high incidence of events during the paramenstruum with incidence varying from 45% to 53% compared with an expected incidence of 29% on an even distribution (Table 5.2) (Dalton 1984). These are days of poorer judgement, lowered resistance to infection, lowered tolerance to pain and decreased visual acuity.

In a survey of emergency hospital admissions due to accidents, it was noted that 52% occurred during the paramenstruum, but there was a marked difference in relation to the parity of the women. In childless women admissions occurred predominantly during the premenstruum and in women who had children admission occurred predominantly during menstruation (Figure 5.3) (Dalton 1960). This difference was not related to marital state, as childless married women tended to be more accident prone during the premenstruum. It was thought to be due to the childless women having a heavy menstrual loss on the first day of menstruation and those who had children having one to three days of slight loss before the full menstrual flow (Dalton 1960).

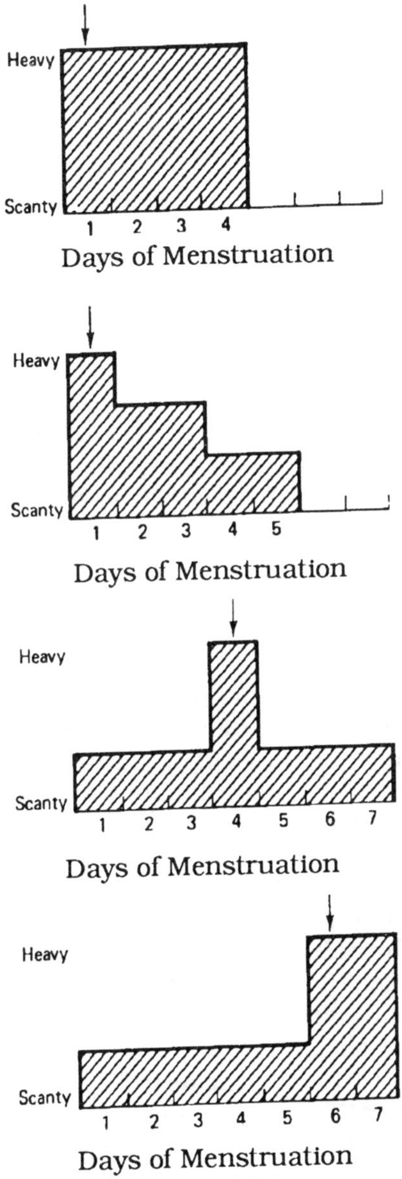

↓ = Relief of premenstrual symptoms.

Figure 5.2 Times of heaviest menstrual flow. *From Dalton K. (1984) 'Premenstrual Syndrome and Progesterone Therapy', 2nd Edition.*

Table 5.2 Events occurring during the paramenstruum: from sociological surveys in North London (Dalton 1977)

	%
Schoolgirls' punishments	45
Industrial employees' sickness	45
Acute psychiatric admission	46
Prisoners commit crimes	49
Acute hospital admissions	49
Eye symptoms in glaucoma	49
Mothers of children admitted to hospital as emergencies	49
Accident admissions	49
Pyrexia in women requiring home visits	52
Visits to doctors' offices by women with sick children	53
Attempted suicides	53

(Expected incidence on even distribution is 29%)

❑ Complete absence of symptoms in the post-menstruum

For legal purposes and in clinical research there must be a complete absence of symptoms for a minimum of seven consecutive days, although in most women with premenstrual syndrome the absence of symptoms lasts considerably longer, usually up to two or three weeks.

An important feature in the precise definition of the premenstrual syndrome is that it locates the symptoms in that phase of the cycle when progesterone should be present (the luteal phase), and their absence when progesterone is absent in the follicular phase. The most acute symptoms of premenstrual syndrome occur when the level of progesterone is dropping from its peak in the mid-luteal phase. This is of importance in the discussion of the etiological factors in the syndrome and in consideration of the success of progesterone therapy.

Magos and Studd (1984) have suggested the definition of premenstrual syndrome as 'distressing physical and psychological symptoms, not caused by organic disease, which regularly recur during the same phase of each ovarian (or menstrual) cycle, and which significantly regress or disappear

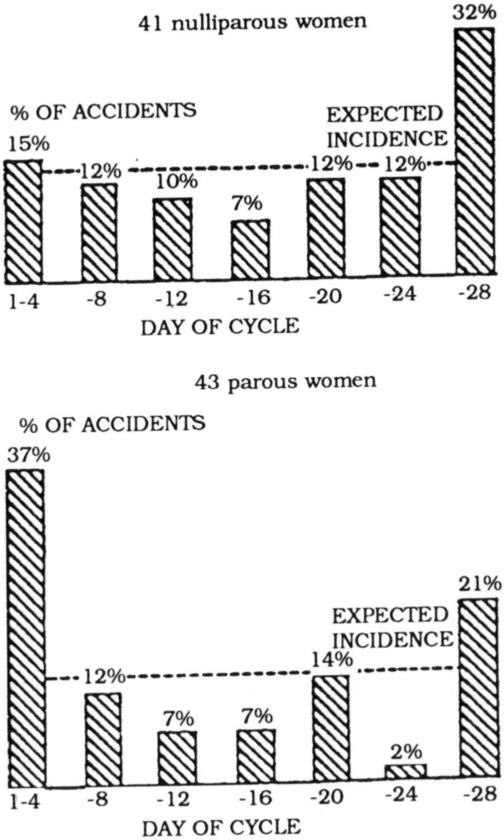

Figure 5.3 Distribution of accidents in nulliparous and parous women. *From Dalton K. (1960) British Medical Journal 2, 1425-1426.*

during the remainder of the cycle'. This definition does require recurrence with each menstrual cycle but it does not require complete absence of symptoms in the postmenstruum.

❑ Irregular menstruation

It has already been mentioned that it is within normal limits for any woman's menstruation to vary by four days month by month. However, those who have irregular menstruation varying by ten or more days each month are unlikely to be suffering from premenstrual syndrome, although they may rightly claim an imbalance of the menstrual hormones.

❑ Menstrual distress

It is important to differentiate premenstrual syndrome from menstrual distress.

'Menstrual distress is the presence of symptoms throughout the menstrual cycle which are worse during the paramenstruum'.

It will be appreciated that this definition does not require recurrent symptoms nor does it demand the complete absence of symptoms in the postmenstruum, thus completely differentiating it from premenstrual syndrome. It is in fact a very vague definition, particularly when it is appreciated that all chronic diseases tend to become worse during the paramenstruum. This includes symptoms which occur only intermittently, such as migraine and epilepsy, as well as continuous symptoms such as occur in multiple sclerosis, rheumatoid or osteo arthritis, bronchitis and glaucoma.

❑ Menstrual distress is not premenstrual syndrome

It is important to appreciate the differences between menstrual distress and premenstrual syndrome, for only the latter is fully responsive to progesterone therapy and only thereby acceptable for legal purposes. *The mere coincidence of a crime being committed during the premenstrual days does not constitute premenstrual syndrome.*

> A 39 year old mother of two children was charged at Wilmslow, Cheshire, with dangerous driving, having been seen to hit a lamppost, mount the kerb twice and drive along the footpath for several yards.
>
> Although the offence occurred during the premenstruum, no further evidence was offered that she suffered from premenstrual syndrome. It could well have been merely a coincidence that it occurred during the premenstruum, and she was duly fined.

The surveys demonstrating the correlation of specified events in relation to menstruation, as shown in Table 5.2, are recording instances of menstrual distress and not premenstrual syndrome. There was no evidence of recurrence of events nor absence in the postmenstruum.

❑ Premenstrual Tension

Premenstrual tension is *'the recurrence of* ***psychological*** *symptoms during the premenstruum with absence in the postmenstruum'*. It will be noted that this definition defines the type of symptoms, whereas the term premenstrual syndrome includes both psychological and somatic symptoms. The common tension symptoms are depression, lethargy and irritability, whereas the somatic or physical symptoms cover disorders of all the organs of the body. (See chapter 8 on symptoms).

Premenstrual tension will also respond to progesterone therapy.

❑ References

Asso D. (1978). *Brit. J. Soc. Clin; Psychol* **17**, 47-55.

Dalton K. (1960). *Brit. Med. J 2,* **1** 425-1 426

Dalton K. (1982). *Behaviour and the Menstrual Cycle.* Ed R.C. Friedman, Marcel Dekker Inc., New York, Chapter 11, 217–242.

Dalton K. (1984). *Premenstrual Syndrome and Progesterone Therapy* 2nd Edition, William Heinemann Medical Books Ltd., London.

Megos A., Studd J. (1984). *Progress in Obstetrics and Gynaecology* **4**, 334–350.

6

Diagnosis of Premenstrual Syndrome

Premenstrual syndrome is the recurrence of symptoms in the premenstruum with complete absence of symptoms in the postmenstruum.

This precise diagnosis is essential in any woman who is pleading premenstrual syndrome in court. The three essentials are:

1. The symptoms that caused the offence had been recurrent, and had been present in at least the last three menstrual cycles.
2. The incident occurred in the premenstruum. This means it occurred before menstruation, usually within a day or two of the onset of menstruation, but at the very longest it cannot occur more than 14 days before menstruation, as that is the time from ovulation to menstruation.
3. There must be complete normality and freedom from symptoms during the postmenstruum.

Symptoms of premenstrual syndrome can either be psychological and/or physical. The actual symptoms, which may give rise to a conflict with the law are discussed in Chapters 8, 9 and 10. The symptoms of premenstrual syndrome must be related to the offence. For instance, it is of no value to produce evidence that the acne on the face, or ulcers in the mouth always occur premenstrually.

In the majority of cases where the woman is pleading premenstrual syndrome the diagnosis must be made retrospectively. Ideally, although it rarely happens, the defendant will be able to produce a menstrual chart, such as is used in many premenstrual syndrome clinics, on which the woman has marked down the symptoms on the day they occur, together with the days of menstruation. The woman is advised to complete her entry each night before retiring. The correlation of symptoms with menstruation and the absence of symptoms in the postmenstruum can be seen at a glance (Figure 6.1).

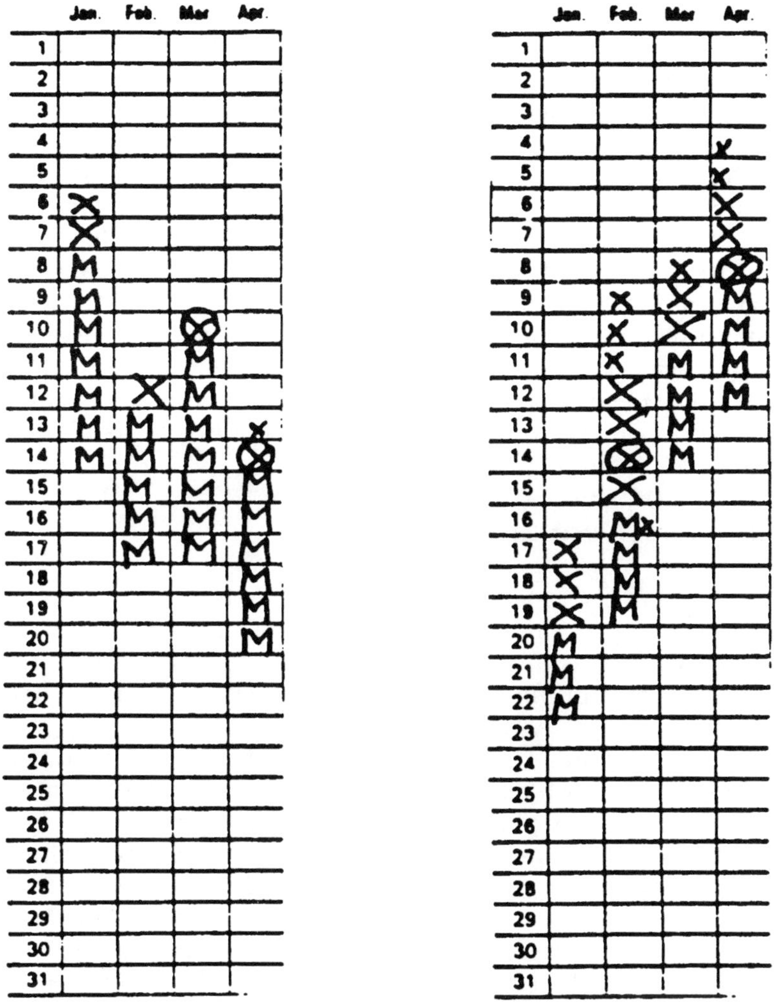

M = menstruation x, X = symptoms, mild or severe

⊗ = offence

Figure 6.1 Menstrual charts recording days of symptoms

From the very beginning of my work on premenstrual syndrome in 1948 it was obvious that some simple, but meticulously accurate, method of recording the timing of symptoms was essential. At the National Hospital for Nervous Diseases, Queens Square, London, a simple chart was in use for marking epileptic attacks. It provided the perfect answer and has been in constant use ever since as the most valuable tool for diagnosing premenstrual syndrome. The chart has now been reduced in size to fit easily into the pocket of a handbag, and is familiarly known as a 'menstrual chart'. Divisions on the chart provide a space for every day of the year from 1st January to 31st December. The patient fills in the chart by marking the symptom in the appropriate space for that month on the day that it occurs, using agreed symbols identifying the premenstrual symptoms and likewise the days of menstruation. This will show clearly the timing of symptoms in relation to menstruation, so confirming or renouncing the diagnosis of premenstrual syndrome.

❑ Questionnaires

There are many questionnaires available, which psychiatrists and others use for the diagnosis and for clinical trials into various treatments for premenstrual syndrome, but these have no place in the retrospective diagnosis of premenstrual syndrome.

The most popular of these is the Moos Menstrual Distress Questionnaire, which was designed to demonstrate the proportion of various populations suffering from menstrual distress, so it includes spasmodic dysmenorrhoea, endometriosis, pelvic inflammatory diseases and other diseases which exacerbate in the paramenstruum. It was not designed to differentiate premenstrual syndrome, nor can it do so. The Moos Menstrual Distress Questionnaire has 47 different questions the woman is expected to complete each night on a six point scale from 'no reaction at all' to 'acute, or partially disabling'. It asks about feelings of loneliness, orderliness, lowered judgement, forgetfulness, restlessness and confusion. It cannot be answered by a woman who is temporarily muddled, confused or amnesic, nor does it ask the relevant questions. 'Did you steal today?', 'Did you hit anyone today?' or 'Did you set fire to anything today?'

Tragic consequences may result from the total reliance on the Moos Menstrual Questionnaire without any consideration of the individual woman crying out for help for her premenstrual syndrome.

> In February 1982 I received a letter from a desperate husband whose wife suffered from premenstrual syndrome with 'raging arguments, tears and numerous symptoms', who had only received ineffective treatment. I replied that she was fortunate in that there was a Premenstrual Syndrome Clinic at the local hospital in her home town, and I suggested she asked her doctor for the necessary letter of referral. J. H. attended the hospital on four occasions, seeing the deputy on the first three. Initially she was given the Moos Menstrual Distress Questionnaire to complete, and then she received progesterone suppositories with marked improvement. She was then given three months without medication to 'see if her body would produce the hormones'. Finally on her fourth visit on 26th June 1983 she saw the consultant psychiatrist, who looked at her questionnaire and felt she suffered from depression in addition to premenstrual syndrome, so refused progesterone. J. H. pleaded unsuccessfully to be allowed to have progesterone, and according to her hospital notes she is reputed to have said "If you don't agree it's hormones and give me treatment which is NOT dummy I'll be six foot under". On lst July 1983, in her premenstruum, she murdered her six year old daughter by stabbing her with scissors, and then tried unsuccessfully to kill herself by stabbing herself with scissors over 200 times, and finally tried running in front of a car. She was injured, but survived in intensive care. Police found all the letters and articles about progesterone on the table in her sitting room. She received a probation order conditional on receiving inpatient treatment for six months and continuation of hormone therapy.

Retrospective questionnaires have no place in the diagnosis of premenstrual syndrome, especially not in women anxious to claim mitigation in law. The conference in Philadelphia referred to at the commencement of Chapter 4, declared in their summary report

> 'Psychological research shows clearly that using

self–reports results in biases of various sorts'.

Sampson and Jenner (1977) have described a method of analysing the data from the Moos Menstrual Distress questionnaires by using sine waves to assess quantitatively the data from the questionnaires, while this differentiates the degree of severity of symptoms in the premenstruum compared with the postmenstruum, it does not differentiate premenstrual syndrome from menstrual distress.

Another example of a questionnaire is the Keith assessment of menstrual symptoms (KAMS) which suggests 30 possible symptoms and asks the woman to note each night the absence or presence of symptoms and to grade each symptom according to severity (Keith1983). This is a useful tool for clinical trials and effectively differentiates premenstrual syndrome from menstrual distress. However if the woman requires retrospective evidence that at the time of the offence she was suffering from premenstrual syndrome the KAMS will not provide the evidence as it was designed for prospective use. It also cannot be used during the paramenstruum by those with psychosis.

The same applies to the use of daily weighing charts or basal temperature charts. The symptoms of premenstrual syndrome, which may be responsible for an offence, will not be demonstrated by such methods.

❑ Diagnostic pointers

The diagnosis of premenstrual syndrome depends on evidence of the correlation of symptoms before menstruation with absence of symptoms in the postmenstruum. However, there are some useful diagnostic pointers from which a checklist score of risk factors can be obtained, and which indicate the woman most at risk and most likely to produce a positive menstrual chart at a later date. This involves careful history taking at the first interview.

❑ Time of onset and increased severity

Premenstrual syndrome tends to start and to increase in severity at those times in a woman's life when marked changes in hormone levels are occurring. Characteristically these take place at puberty, following a pregnancy, during or after using the contraceptive pill, after some months without menstruation, after removal of one ovary, and following sterilisation. In a series of 1,095 women with severe premenstrual syndrome requiring progesterone therapy 87% reported the onset of symptoms following one of these hormonal events, and 86% reported increased severity following such hormonal events. (Dalton 1984) (Table 6.1).

Table 6.1 Time of Onset and Increased Severity of Premenstrual Syndrome

n = 1095

	Onset	Increased Severity
	%	%
Hormonal Event	87	86
Non-hormonal Event	9	14
Unknown	4	-
Puberty	32	-
After Abortion	-	3
After Pregnancy	33	49
After Postnatal Depression	8	9
Oral Contraceptives	8	10
After Amenorrhoea	3	4
After Sterilisation	3	11
After Oophorectomy	1	-

❑ Painless menstruation

Painless menstruation is a characteristic feature of severe premenstrual syndrome and is often the very reason why sufferers of psychosis, epilepsy, migraine and asthma fail to make the connection. Occasionally, there may be increasing continuous lower abdominal pain, bloatedness and heaviness occurring in the premenstruum which eases with menstruation and is known as 'congestive dysmenorrhoea'. However spasmodic dysmenorrhoea, in which the young woman curls up with colicky abdominal pain at the onset of menstruation and may even vomit or faint, is rare in premenstrual syndrome.

The shoplifter who claimed her period pains were so severe that she was under the influence of analgesics was really suffering from spasmodic dysmenorrhoea and not from premenstrual syndrome which she pleaded in mitigation.

❑ Increase in libido in the premenstruum

Increased libido, or sex urge, in adolescents and childless women is frequent and is responsible for some young adolescents being made wards of court when their parents can no longer control their episodic running away from home. It does not occur after postnatal depression. It is seen in those 'good' daughters who come home each night at the time the parents requested, except on their premenstrual day when they stay out all night harassing the boys. If committed to a children's home or detention centre they still run away each premenstruum.

Among those who have reported this increased premenstrual libido, occasionally reaching nymphomanic proportions are Israel (1983), Gray (1941) and Hart (1960). Shader and his colleagues (1968) studied the changes in libido throughout the menstrual cycle in 76 female graduates and noted that the premenstrual increase was most marked in anxious women (58%) ($P = <0.01$) and in those of higher social groups ($P = <0.05$). This increased libido distinguishes premenstrual syndrome from a depressive illness in which there is a decrease in libido throughout the cycle.

❑ Inability to tolerate the oral contraceptive

Women with premenstrual syndrome have difficulty in tolerating oral contraceptives. They are the ones who change brands and finally stop because of depression, headaches, weight gain and increased tension. Among 614 women with premenstrual syndrome, 85% had side effects on the pill (Dalton 1984). (Fig 6.2) This is in contrast to those women with spasmodic dysmenorrhoea, menorrhagia or irregular menstruation who positively benefit from oral contraceptives.

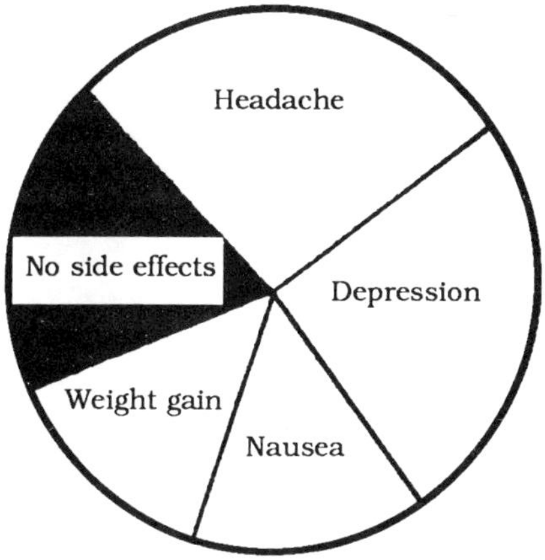

Figure 6.2 Side effects of oral contraceptives in Premenstrual Syndrome

The artificial progestogens, which are an essential component of all contraceptive pills are generally 19-nor-testosterone derivatives, their formulae is closer to that of testosterone than of progesterone (Figure 6.3). Artificial progestogens, which are alien to the human body, should not be confused with natural progesterone, some of their properties are quite different. For example, progesterone administration raises the blood progesterone level, while progestogens lower the blood progesterone level. Progesterone raises SHBG levels, whereas progestogens lower SHBG levels. Progesterone administration may lower the blood pressure, but progestogens may cause a rise in the blood pressure. Premenstrual syndrome appears to be related to a deficiency of progesterone, and it is not surprising that sufferers of premenstrual syndrome have difficulty in tolerating drugs which reduce their progesterone level.

Unfortunately many young girls are prescribed oral contraceptives when their premenstrual anti-social behaviour is first noticed, but such treatment only results in further deterioration.

❑ Weight fluctuation in adult life

All women, in contrast to men, have twice monthly weight swings. In sufferers of premenstrual syndrome this may exceed the normal 4-5 lbs. If one compares a woman's highest-

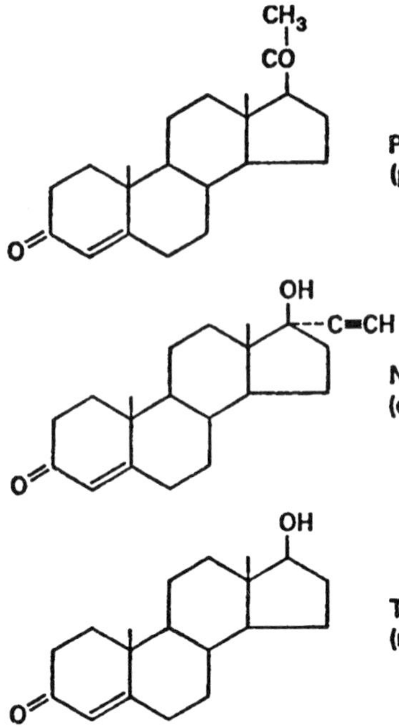

Progesterone
(pregnancy hormone)

Norethisterone
(oral contraceptive)

Testosterone
(male hormone)

Figure 6.3 Which compound does norethisterone resemble?

ever non–pregnant weight with her lowest-ever weight since she left school, it will be noticed that women with premenstrual syndrome often experience an adult weight swing of over 28 lbs. This is noticed more often among women who first attend for consultation at the average age of 35 years, rather than those involved in legal problems who tend to be in the younger age group.

❑ Altered hunger tolerance

Sufferers of premenstrual syndrome cannot tolerate long intervals without food and are liable to develop acute symptoms of irritability, violence, fainting or panic attacks after going for 5 or more hours during the day without food. They may complain that their lives consist of episodes of strict dieting and fasting followed by uncontrolled cravings and binges (Smith & Saunder 1968). It is important to take a full history of the times and type of all food eaten on the day of an alleged incident. The importance of the advice to eat frequent small amounts of carbohydrates and the reason for it is contained in Chapters 11 and 12.

❑ Effect of pregnancy

During pregnancy there is an immediate rise in the blood levels of progesterone which finally reach some fifty times the level present at the mid-luteal peak (page 22). This means that sufferers of premenstrual syndrome lose their symptoms during pregnancy. Comments of some of these women with severe premenstrual syndrome, speaking about their pregnancy, include: 'absolutely wonderful – never better', 'happiest ever.... for the first time I knew normal health', 'placid.... sweet.... reading again'. However, there is a high incidence of threatened abortion (bleeding during early pregnancy) and of pre-eclampsia (raised blood pressure, swelling of the ankles and protein in the urine). The incidence of premenstrual syndrome after pre-eclampsia (toxaemia) is high, 87% after one pregnancy and rising to 100% after four pregnancies (Dalton 1954). Among sufferers of premenstrual syndrome there is also a high incidence of postnatal depression, severe enough to require medical treatment. In one recent survey of 769 sufferers of premenstrual syndrome, as many as 59% developed postnatal depression compared with 14% normal population (Dalton 1984). Among 300 women, all of whom had suffered from postnatal depression, as many as 86% subsequently developed premenstrual syndrome (Dalton 1985) (Figure 6.4). All of which reveals a close relationship between threatened abortion, pre-eclampsia, postnatal depression and premenstrual syndrome.

❑ Diagnostic checklist score

The items mentioned in the list of diagnostic pointers (Table 6.2) can be scored 'positive', 'negative' and 'non-relevant' and the checklist score calculated as follows:

$$\text{Diagnostic checklist score} = \frac{\text{Positives} \times 100}{\text{Positives} + \text{Negatives}}$$

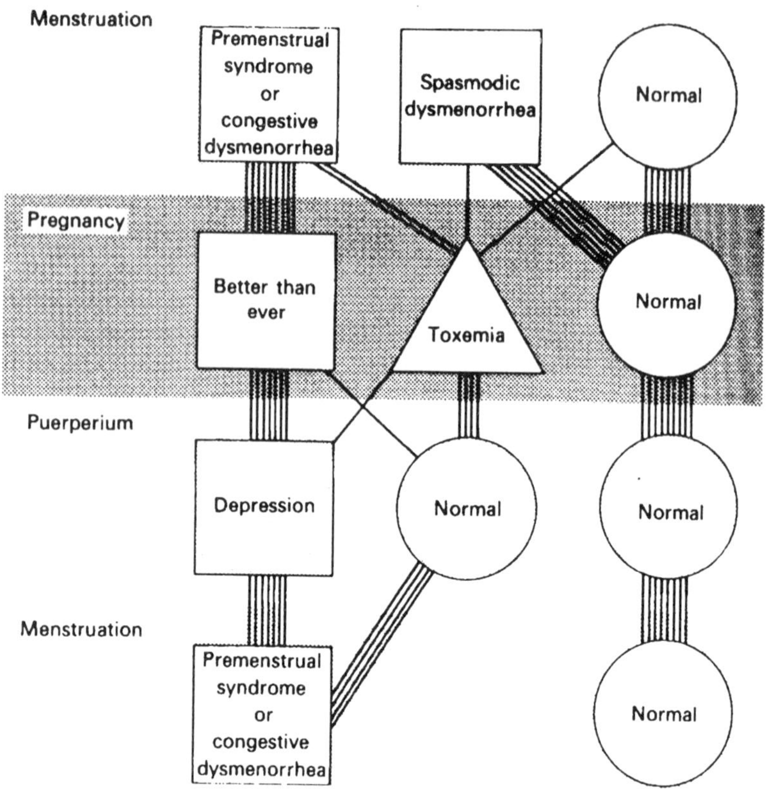

Figure 6.4 Effect of pregnancy on menstruation. *From Dalton K. (1969), The Menstrual Cycle, Penguin Books.*

Table 6.2 Diagnostic Pointers

	Non relevant	Positive	Negative	
Time of onset				
Time of increased severity				
Painless menstruation				
Increased libido in premenstruum (childless women only)				
Threatened abortion				
Pre-eclampsia				
Postnatal depression				
Side effects with the Pill				
Adult weight swings over 2 stone				
Altered hunger tolerance				in premenstruum
Altered alcohol tolerance				in premenstruum

Items scored 'non-relevant', are omitted. Such items might include the effect of the pill on a non-user, complications of pregnancy in one who has not been pregnant and altered food tolerance in one who had not previously considered this possibility. (Table 6.2). A diagnostic checklist score of 66% or more is most likely to produce a positive menstrual chart at a later date. A diagnostic checklist score of 100% is important, but nevertheless, it is not a positive diagnosis without the evidence of a menstrual chart. (Dalton 1982). Figure 6.5 portrays the high incidence of those risk factors which have been demonstrated in surveys.

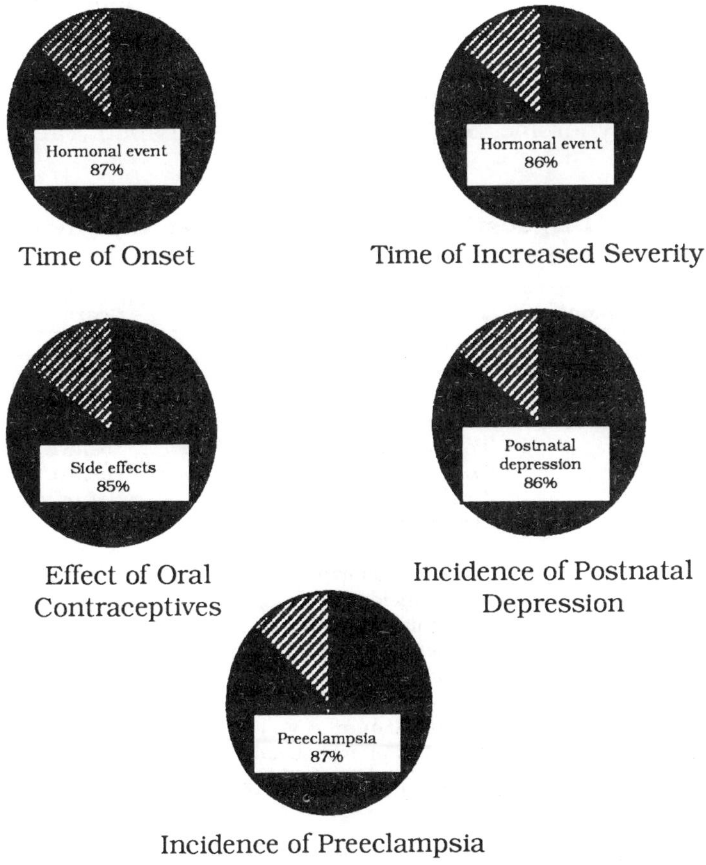

Figure 6.5 Diagnostic pointers for premenstrual syndrome

❑ Legal application of a diagnostic checklist score

The medical records of C. E., a mother of two who was charged with fatally injuring her lover, demonstrated clearly that she suffered from premenstrual syndrome and had twice been admitted in the premenstruum with suicide attempts. She had twice suffered from postnatal depression requiring hospital admission and was unable to tolerate the pill. During her stay in the police cell immediately after the incident she had commented to the police about her increased libido premenstrually. She started menstruating 19 hours after the incident while in the police cell. Her diagnostic checklist score of 100% was presented in court and accepted as evidence of premenstrual syndrome. She was released on probation (Table 6.3).

Table 6.3 Diagnostic pointers in 34 year old divorced mother of two children charged with murder

Diagnostic pointer	History	Score
Onset	First Pregnancy	Positive
Increased severity	Second pregnancy	Positive
	Sterilisation	Positive
Painless menstruation	Painless	Positive
Pregnancy	Postnatal Depression x 2	Positive x 2
Pill	Loss of Libido	Positive
Weight swing	Unable to recall	Not relevant
Hunger	Recognised unable to tolerate food gaps 9 hours food gap before incident	Positive
Alcohol	Recognised inability to tolerate premenstrually and abstained	Positive
Libido	Increased in the premenstruum	Positive
Incident	19 hours premenstrual	Positive
	Diagnostic checklist score = 100%	

In 1981, S.N., a 33 year old mother of two children, was charged with infanticide. She drowned her three month baby and then took a massive overdose. The mother was resuscitated, but the baby died. The incident occurred the day before menstruation. She had eaten no food since 0800 hours and is thought to have drowned the baby at 1700 hours. Perusal of her medical records showed that she had received treatment for premenstrual syndrome from puberty until the birth of her first child. Her first pregnancy had been complicated by pre-eclampsia and her second was followed by postnatal depression for which she received psychiatric treatment. In her early twenties she was unable to tolerate the pill which caused such a high rise in her blood pressure that she was admitted to the London Hospital for investigations. She recognised she became bad-tempered after long intervals without food. She abstained from alcohol.Her diagnostic checklist score was 100%. She was successful in her plea of premenstrual syndrome and released on probation. She had a daughter weighing 8lbs in August 1983, and received progesterone prophylaxis for postnatal depression. Both mother and daughter are presently in excellent health, and their names have been removed from the At Risk Register. (Table 6.4).

Table 6.4 Diagnostic pointers in 33 year old mother of two children charged with infanticide

Diagnostic pointer	History	Score
Onset	Puberty	Positive
Increased severity	After first pregnancy	Positive
Painless menstruation	Yes	Positive
Pregnancy	First pre-eclampsia	Positive
	Second postnatal depression	Positive
Pill	Raised blood pressure	Positive
Weight swing	30lbs in adult life	Positive
Hunger	Binges premenstrually	Positive
Alcohol	Abstained	Not Relevant
Incident	24 hours premenstrually	Positive
	Diagnostic checklist score = 100%	

It must be appreciated that in America such comprehensive medical notes are often unavailable, and this makes retrospective diagnosis more difficult.

❑ Biochemical tests

There is little diagnostic value to be obtained from radioimmunoassay of progesterone in the luteal phase, nor of oestradiol, FSH, LH or prolactin, although serial estimations of these hormones for research purposes in premenstrual syndrome sufferers and normal controls, one day may help to unravel aetiological factors. Premenstrual syndrome can occur in women who are not ovulating; but since all women who are not ovulating do not suffer from premenstrual syndrome, a low progesterone level at the mid luteal phase is not helpful in diagnosis.

❑ Sex Hormone Binding Globulin

Hormones are chemical messengers, they are made in one organ and have an action on some distant tissue. The menstrual hormones, progesterone and oestrogen, are made in the ovaries, but their action is not limited to the womb. Oestrogen is also required by the breasts, bones and skin, whereas progesterone is also required by brain cells, eyes, skin and the nasopharyngeal passages and the lungs. The sex hormones are transported round the body in the blood attached, or bound, to minute protein molecules called globulins. It is possible to measure the binding capacity of sex hormone binding globulin or SHBG. A series of fifty women suffering from severe premenstrual syndrome were found to have SHBG levels below the average of 50 – 80 nmol/1, when compared with a group of fifty healthy women, who on direct questioning stated they did not suffer from premenstrual syndrome (Dalton M. 1981) (Figure 6.6).

The SHBG estimation is a specialised test, which is not done routinely and only in a few specialised centres in Britain. The blood sample must be collected, centrifuged and stored frozen until analysed.The women to be tested must be free from all medications, including the pill, sedatives, analgesics, and herbal tablets; be free from thyroid or liver disease; must not be obese; nor be unduly hirsute; and this proscription includes some women of the ethnically hirsute races. SHBG can be estimated any day of the menstrual cycle.

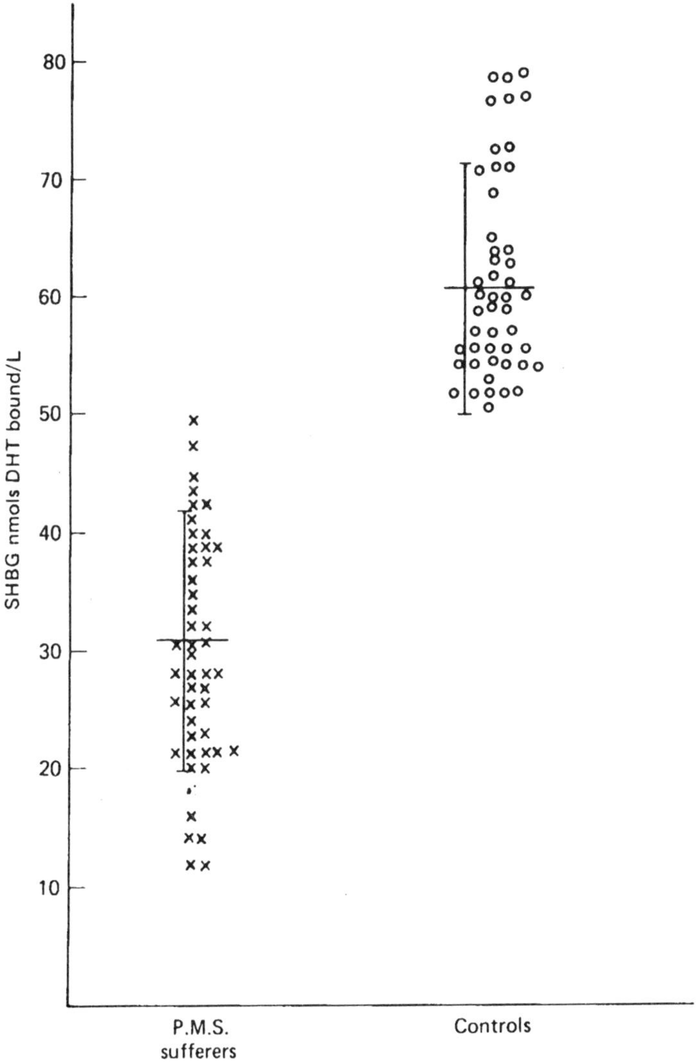

Figure 6.6 SHBG-binding capacity in 50 patients with severe premenstrual syndrome compared with 50 controls. *From Dalton K. (1984) 'Premenstrual Syndrome and Progesterone Therapy', 2nd Edition.*

It is not known why the SHBG is low in premenstrual syndrome, but it is interesting that when progesterone is given there is a dose responsive rise in SHBG level (Dalton M, 1984) (Figure 6.7). Conversely, when the artificial progestogens are given the SHBG is lowered. Progestogens make premenstrual syndrome worse and they also lower the blood progesterone level.

An SHBG estimation may be valuable evidence of the presence of premenstrual syndrome, but it is essential to comply with the necessary requirements for estimation.

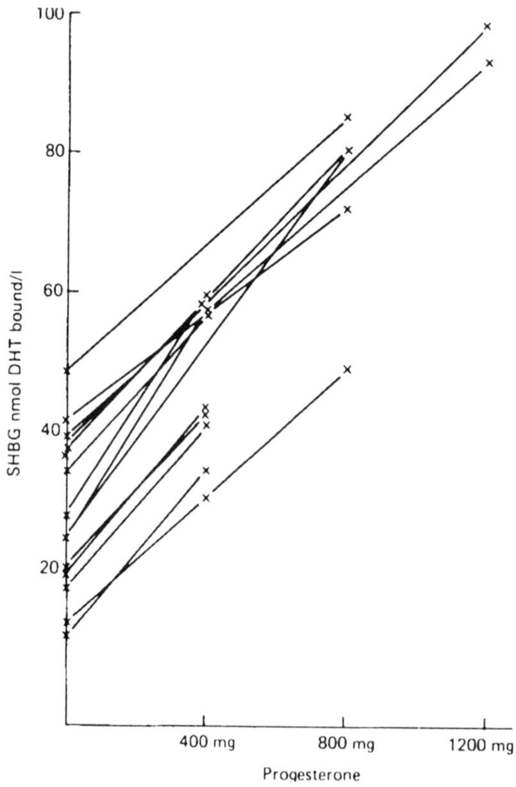

Figure 6.7 Effect of progesterone on SHBG levels. *From Dalton K. (1984) 'Premenstrual Syndrome and Progesterone Therapy', 2nd Edition.*

A.R. appealed against her life sentence for murder and a request was made to collect a blood sample for an SHBG test. All medication was stopped for the required seven days and she was sent down from Durham prison to Holloway prison in London for examination and the collection of her blood sample. Unfortunately the request for the blood sample had not been correctly received by the principal medical office, and following her examination she was sent back to Durham and medication resumed. After a further seven days without medication a pathologist took the necessary sample, which was then transported by Securicor to the London laboratories where it was analysed. Her SHBG was very low at 14, compared with the normal 50–80 nmol/l, and formed important evidence. She was freed on two years probation.

❑ Comparison of diagnostic checklist score and SHBG

A correlation of the effectiveness of a diagnostic checklist score with SHBG estimation is shown in a scattergram in Figure 6.8 (Dalton 1984). Sixty five women were referred to the premenstrual clinic by their general practitioners with a presumed diagnosis of premenstrual syndrome. On examination, only 42 (65%) had the diagnosis confirmed by a three month menstrual chart. The remaining 35% had some other diagnosis to account for their symptoms.

In a further study, 256 women similarly referred for premenstrual syndrome were grouped three months later according to the result of their menstrual charts. Premenstrual syndrome was diagnosed in 112 women (42%) in the PMS group, a double diagnosis was present in 42 women who were excluded from the study, and 102 women showed no correlation of symptoms with the timing of their menstruation and were placed in the non-PMS group. There was no age difference between the various groups. The diagnostic checklist score was elevated in 83% of the PMS group and 60% of the non-PMS group ($P = <0.004$). The only risk items found significantly more often in the PMS group were:

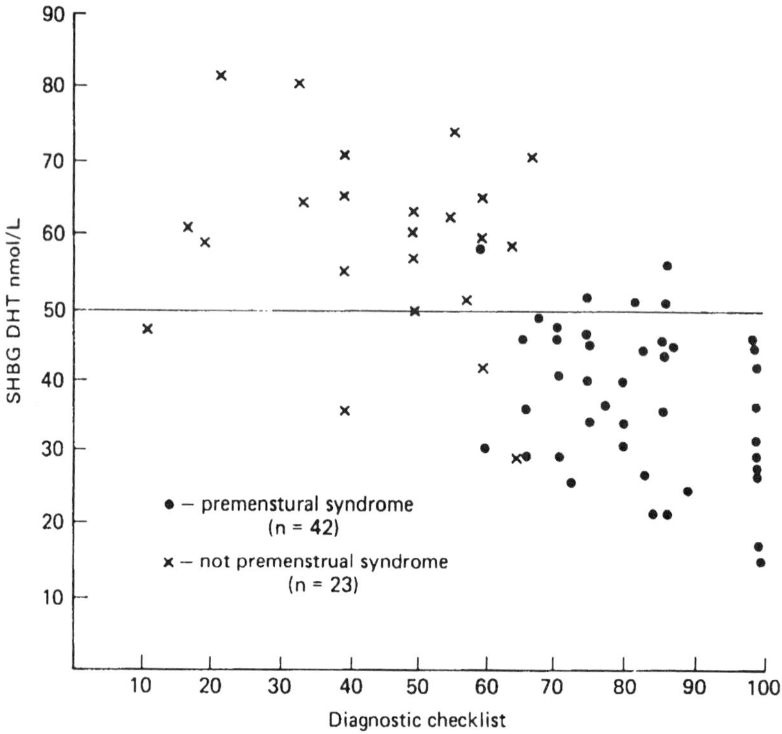

Figure 6.8 Scattergram of SHBG and diagnostic checklist percentage. *From Dalton K. (1984) 'Premenstrual Syndrome and Progesterone Therapy', 2nd Edition*

1. an adult weight swing exceeding 28 lbs,
2. side effects on oral contraceptives
3. a history of postnatal depression.

The SHBG was low in 87% of the PMS group compared with 39% of the non-PMS group (P = <0.001). Comparison showed SHBG to be more specific, more sensitive and to have a higher predictive value than the diagnostic checklist score. (Dalton & Dalton 1985).

❑ References

Dalton K. (1984). *Premenstrual Syndrome and Progesterone Therapy 2nd Ed.;* William Heinemann Medical Books Ltd., London/Year Book Publications Inc., Chicago.
Dalton K. and Dalton M.E. (1985). *Int. Cong. Psychosom. Obst. & Gynaec.*, Vienna
Dalton M.E. (1981). *Postgrad. Med. J.;* **57**, 560-562
Dalton M.E. (1984). *J. Ster. Biochem.;* Jan.
Hart R.S. (1960). Brit. Med. J.; **1**, 1023.
lqbal M.J. & Johnston (1977). *J. Ster. Biochem.;* **8**, 977-85
Israel S.L. (1983). *Brit. Med. J.;* **110**, 1721
Keith G. (1983). *Personal Communication.*
Moos R. (1983). *Psychosom. Med.;* **30**, 853-867
Sampson G.A. & Jenner F.A. (1977). *Brit J. Psychiat.;* 103, 256-271
Shader R.I., Mascio A. & Harmatz J. (1968). *Psychosomat.;* **9**. 197-198
Smith S. & Saunder C. (1969). *Psychosom. Med.;* 31, 4., 281.

7

Behaviour and Menstruation

The physicians of the Hippocratic era recognised the tension that preceded menstruation and attributed this to 'the agitated blood trying to find a way out of the woman's body'. They also noted that 'shivering, lassitude and heaviness of the head denotes the onset of menstruation 'and that 'mistiness of vision is resolved by the onset of menstruation'. (Magog and Studd 1984).

Simonides in his 'Essay on Woman' wrote in 6th Century B.C.

> "She has two different sorts of mood. One day she is all smiles and happiness.Then another day there will be no living with her, you can't get within sight, or come near her, or she flies into a rage and holds you at a distance like a bitch with pups, cantankerous and cross with all the World ... The sea is like that also. Often it lies calm and innocent and still ... Then it will go wild and turbulent... This woman's disposition is just like the sea's since the sea's temper also changes all the time".
>
> *(Lloyd Jones 1978)*

This quotation merely serves to remind us that the mood swings so characteristic of a woman's behaviour are not new. Indeed the many myths surrounding menstruation, which exist worldwide, suggest that the intermittent antisocial behaviour of women may have been even more marked in the ancient world than it is today.

In the search for examples of crime associated with menstruation, one needs to recall Martha Brixley, who in 1845 murdered her employer's child. There was an absence of motive and no attempt to escape the consequences of her act. She was acquitted on the plea of insanity due to 'obstructed menstruation,' and was apparently receiving treatment for her amenorrhoea (Smith 1981). In 1845, Ann Shepher was charged at Carlisle Quarter Sessions for stealing a fur boa, and also acquitted on the grounds of 'temporary insanity from suppression of the menses'. In 1851 Amelia Snoswell was charged at Maidstone Assizes with murdering her baby niece, and also acquitted on the grounds of insanity due to disordered menstruation (D'Orban 1983). But these crimes all occurred in the days before massive media exposure.

D'Orban (1983) quoted Lombroso and Ferrero (1894) among the first criminologists to observe antisocial behaviour associated with menstruation when they reported 80 women arrested for 'resistance to public officials', of whom 71 (89%) were menstruating. Previously Icard (1890) studied 56 Parisian shoplifters of whom 35 (62.5%) were menstruating at the time of their offence. French figures showed that 84% of crimes of violence by women were committed during or immediately before menstruation (Cooke 1945). Morton *et al* (1953) in New York found that of 42 women sentenced for crimes of violence, 62% had committed their crimes during the premenstrual week.

In 1961 a London survey into 156 women who were regularly menstruating and had all committed their crime in the preceding 28 days found that 49% ($P =< 0.001$) had committed their crime during the paramenstruum, defined as the last four days before menstruation or the first four days of menstruation. (Dalton 1961). Premenstrual syndrome was present in 27% of the 156 newly convicted prisoners, and in these it was noted that 63% had committed their crimes during the paramenstruum. The dates of conviction of a further 102 women who were menstruating regularly but whose crime had been committed more than 28 days previously were evenly distributed throughout the cycle suggesting that menstruation had no prejudicial effect on those women during their court appearance.

Ninety four prisoners, whose bad behaviour was reported to the prison governor, were also studied and 54% were found to be disorderly during their paramenstruum. Among 54 prisoners reported only once for bad behaviour, 43% of the offences were committed in the paramenstruum compared with 70% who were reported more than once.

In 1980 D'Orban and Dalton investigated a series of 50 consecutive female admissions, to the same London prison, of women charged with crimes of violence, including 32 charged with violence to the person (including murder, manslaughter, attempted murder, grievous bodily harm and assault) and 18 with violence against property (arson and criminal damage). Forty four percent of the violent offences were committed during the paramenstruum (P = <0.02), and a significant number of the offences occurred on the 28th day (P = <0.005) and the first day (P = <0.02).

There was a marked similarity in the influence of menstruation on the timing of the crime in these two studies conducted in the same prison after a time interval of twenty years (Figure 7.1). The Dalton study covered all crime, including theft, soliciting, drunkenness and violence whereas the study by D'Orban and Dalton was limited to violent crimes.

D'Orban and Dalton further questioned the 50 women about the presence of premenstrual symptoms and found that 17 (34%) reported premenstrual symptoms, the commonest of

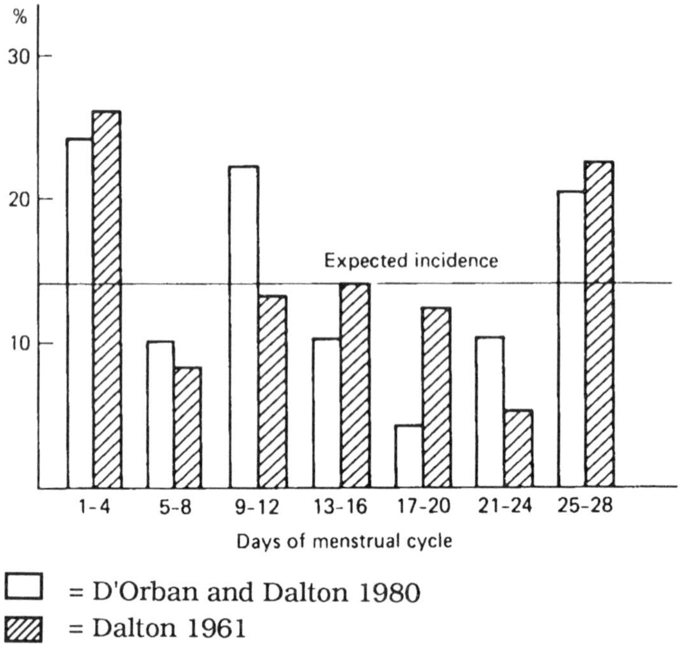

Figure 7.1 Distribution of 50 offences of violence and 156 other offences (Dalton K. 1961) during four-day periods of the menstrual cycle. *From D'Orban P. T. and Dalton J. (1980). Psychological Medicine;* ***10****: 353-359.*

which were depression (14%) and irritability (14%). Only two women thought that menstruation had any influence on the offence charged. This may be compared with the three women described on the first page in the introduction. All were unaware of the effect of their menstruation although it had been recognised by their respective father, but who all were found to have cyclical episodes of violence in the premenstruum (Dalton 1980).

The effect of menstruation on behaviour was also studied at an English boarding school, where it was customary to record in punishment books the date and type of any offence and where it was also normal for the Matron to keep records of the girls' menstruation. During the term under observation 272 offences were committed, of which 29% occurred during the first four days of menstruation. This rate was twice the expected incidence on a normal distribution (P = <0.001). This study also revealed a marked similarity in the effect of menstruation on behaviour in these schoolgirls and the women prisoners previously cited (Figure 7.2).

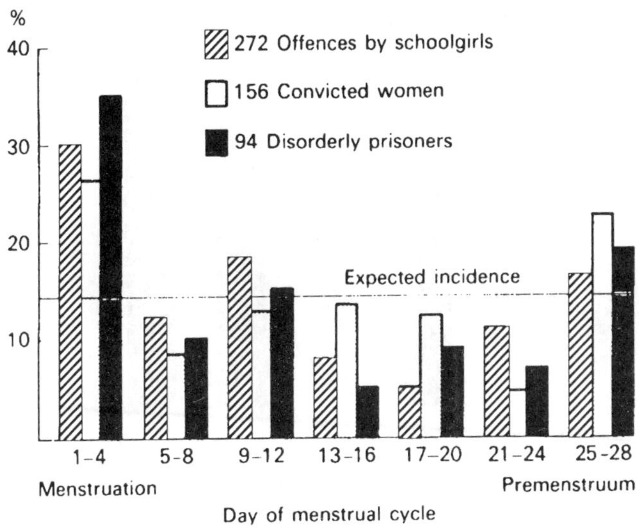

Figure 7.2 Times of offences during menstrual cycle. *From Dalton K. (1961). Br. Med. J.;* ***2****: 1752.*

Offences which predominated during menstruation included unpunctuality, forgetfulness and avoiding games, while talking when silence was requested was less significant as a menstrual offence. Eating during lessons and wearing the wrong clothes occurred evenly throughout the cycle. The 'good' girls with only one or two offences per term committed 26% of their offences during menstruation (as compared with the chance expectation of 14%) whereas, the 'naughty' girls with six or more offences per term were even more influenced by their menstruation, committing 36% of their offences during this four day period (Figure 7.3). The word 'naughty' and 'naughtiness' have been deliberately chosen to avoid more serious associations of a term like 'behaviour disorder'.

Twenty seven girls were selected, all of whom had committed more than four offences during the term, and the headmistress was asked to supply additional details. These girls were then grouped into three categories:

1. behaviour influenced by menstruation, that is more than 50% of their offences were committed during the first four days of menstruation.

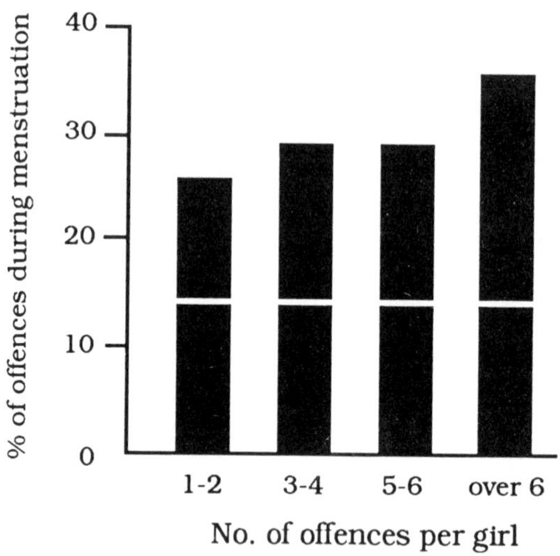

Figure 7.3 Number of offences of schoolgirls per term and those committed during menstruation. *From Dalton K. (1969). British Medical Journal;* ***2****, 1425-1426*

2. behaviour possibly influenced by menstruation, with 25 to 50% of offences committed during menstruation.
3. behaviour not affected by menstruation, that is less than 25% of the offences committed during menstruation.

The headmistress was then shown the three lists of girls without knowing how or why they had been grouped. The nine girls most affected by menstruation were described as 'just naughty from exuberance or laziness'. Three had personal stress, e.g. broken home, ill parent, and the average intelligence of all in this group was high, with only two in the lowest of the three academic streams. Their commonest offence was lateness and talking. They contrasted sharply with the list of eight girls unaffected by menstruation, who were described as 'problem girls requiring careful handling and understanding'. Seven of the eight had personal stress problems, one girl being described as 'the most unfortunate girl in the whole school of 400 children'. Their general level of intelligence was below the average, with five of the eight girls in the lowest stream. Disobedience and rudeness were their commonest offences. This distribution suggested two types of naughtiness in school, physiological due to hormonal changes and psychological naughtiness related to stress. The former was most marked among the brighter, well adjusted girls, whereas the latter was more marked among poor achievers (Dalton 1960).

❑ Critical Event Analysis

The appreciation of the adverse effect of menstruation on schoolgirls and women prisoners raised the question of whether there could be similar behaviour patterns in males. An analysis was made based on the time interval between two documented offences as recorded in boys 'and girls' boarding schools and men's and women's prisons (Dalton 1964). In the women prisoners and the menstruating and premenarcheal schoolgirls the findings were almost identical. If they had offended once they were likely to offend again within the next 4 days; from then on there is a gradual decline until day 25 when a sudden peak occurred until day 28 and then the decline continued (Figure 7.4).

In the schoolboys, the pattern is similar but without the peak

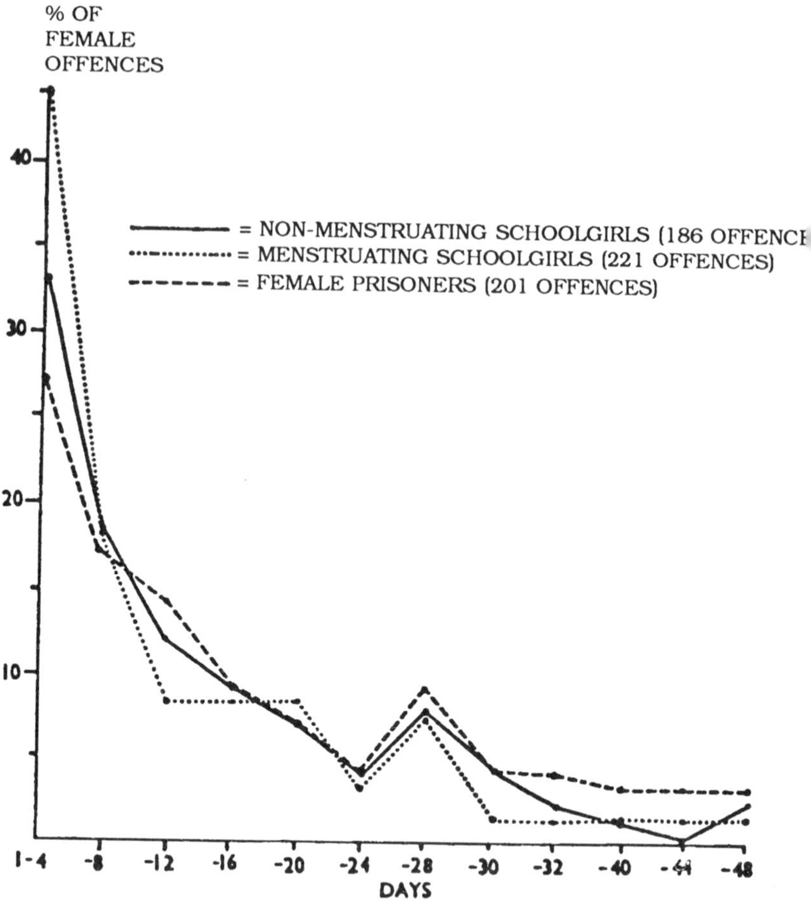

Figure 7.4 Time intervals between offences in females.
From Dalton K. (1964). Proc Roy Soc Med **57**, *4, 18.*

at days 25 to 28. The male prisoners, however, show a slightly different pattern. The highest proportion of recurrences occurred on the 9th to 12th day after the first offence and thereafter gradually declined in a similar pattern to the schoolboys (Figure 7.5).

These observations suggest that although it is possible that a hormonal cycle is also present in males, either such cycles are not marked by periods of lethargy and poor discipline or the male cycle is so irregular that it is imperceptible in an analysis

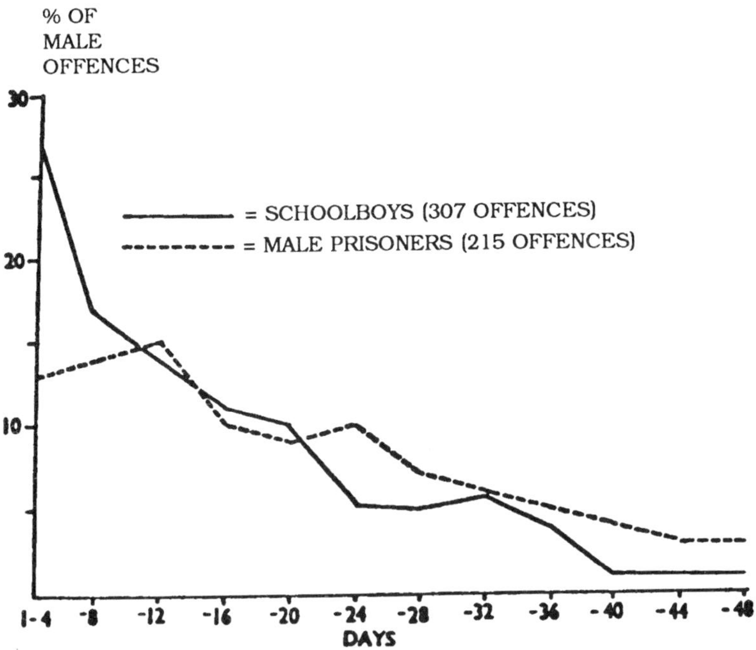

Figure 7.5 Time interval between offences in males. *From Dalton K. (1964). Proc Roy Soc Med* **57***, 4, 18.*

of this type. Incidentally, this critical event analysis has also been conducted in men and women with glaucomatous episodes and with headaches. whereas there is a peak at days 25 to 28 in the females, it is not present in the males (Figure 7.6).

Norris (1983) recalls that during an unreported research project into the aggressive behaviour of women conducted at a Massachusetts prison some years earlier six women sentenced for murder were interviewed. Their victims had been three husbands, two children, and one lover. Two things were striking in regard to all six women: 1) the killings had occurred on the day before or the first day of menstruation and, 2) all six were described as 'quiet, mild mannered housewives'. Norris states that Enid Bagnold observed 'a murderess is only an ordinary woman in a temper', Norris then adds, 'That could be the temper of premenstrual syndrome'.

Further consideration of antisocial behaviour specifically

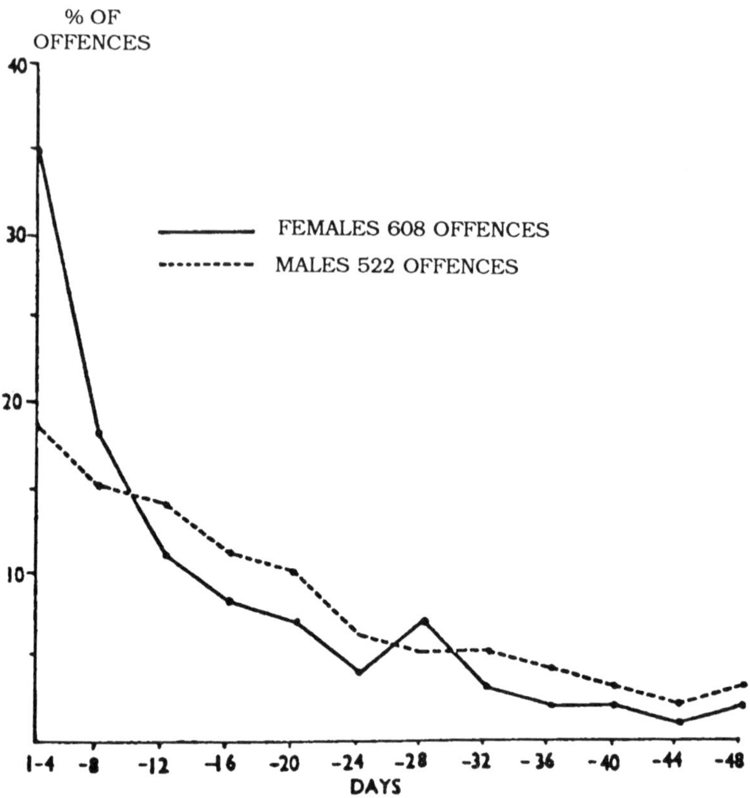

Figure 7.6 Time intervals between offences in males and females. *From Dalton K. (1964). Proc Roy Soc Med* **57**, *4, 18.*

related to premenstrual syndrome is contained in Chapters 9 and 10.

❑ References

Cooke W.R. (1945). *Amer. J. Obstet. Gynec.;* **49**, 475

Dalton K. (1960). *Brit. Med. J.;* **2**, 1647–1649

Dalton K. (1961). *Brit. Med. J.;* **2**, 1752–1753

Dalton K. (1964). *Premenstrual Syndrome;* William Heinemann Medical Books, London.

D'Orban P.T. (1983). *Brit. J. Hosp. Med.;* Dec. 404.

D'Orban P.T. & Dalton J. (1980). *Psychol. Med.;* **10**, 353-359

Morton J.H., Additon H., Addison R.G., Hunt L. & Sullivan J.J. (1953). *Amer. J. Obst. Gynec.;* **65**, 1182-1191.
Norris R.V. & Sullivan C. (1983). *Premenstrual Syndrome;* Rawson Associates, New York.
Smith R. (1981). *Trial by Medicine; Insanity and Responsibility in Victorian Trials;* Edinburgh University Press, Edinburgh.

8

Symptoms causing Premenstrual Syndrome Crimes

Over one hundred and fifty different symptoms have been described which may occur in premenstrual syndrome. The symptoms cover almost every medical speciality and the premenstrual syndrome appears to be amongst the commonest presentations with which each speciality is called upon to deal. Thus, the common symptoms taking women to psychiatrists are depression, irritability, tiredness and tension, the neurologists see most patients complaining of epilepsy, migraine, vertigo and blackouts; the rheumatologists and orthopaedic surgeons see those with backache and vague joint pains; the dermatologists have their appointments filled with women complaining of acne and boils; the chest physicians with those suffering from asthma; the urologists are concerned with recurrent cystitis and urethritis, and the allergists see those complaining of urticaria, rhinitis, asthma and migraine. Nor must one forget those trying to treat the recurrent sore throats, upper respiratory infections and sinusitis. Furthermore, the women with premenstrual syndrome tend to be polysymptomatic, their symptoms often span more than one speciality.

The symptoms of premenstrual syndrome may be conveniently divided into psychological and somatic, but since it is only the psychological symptoms which may be associated with criminal offences, only those will be considered here. It needs to be repeated, however, that not all premenstrual syndrome patients are potential criminals, any more than all criminals are potential sufferers of premenstrual syndrome.

Rubinow and his colleagues (1984) reminded us that as early as 1835 Pritchard described premenstrual syndrome as 'Some females, at the catamenia (menstruation), undergo a considerable degree of nervous excitement; morbid dispositions of mind are displayed by them at these times, a wayward and capricious temper, excitability of feelings, moroseness indisposition, a proneness to quarrel with their nearest relatives, and sometimes a dejection of mind approaching to melancholia'. Icard (1880) observed the following during menstruation: 'kleptomania, pyromania, dipsomania, homicidal mania, suicidal mania, erotomania, nymphomania, delirious insanity, impulsive insanity, morbid, jealousy, lying, calumny, illusions, hallucinations and melancholiia'. All these criminal activities can indeed occur in premenstrual syndrome today, which merely serves to remind us of the skills of clinical observation employed before the era of scientific medicine. Today clinical observation is apt to be regarded by the scientists as anecdotal, and its importance is often disregarded by these individuals. Indeed, older clinicians sometimes wonder if their younger counterparts are not missing some important facts in their total reliance on laboratory medicine.

The commonest premenstrual syndrome symptoms, as mentioned in the popular press, are tension, breast tenderness, bloatedness, headache and backache, however, it is premenstrual tension with its triad of components, 'depression, irritability and lethargy', which most frequently results in conflict with the law. Other rarely mentioned symptoms which may have legal consequences are temporary psychosis (with confusion, delusions, hallucinations or paranoia) and nymphomania.

❑ Depression

Medical students are taught that the typical type of depressive illness is 'a disease of loss', for there is loss of happiness, pleasure, interests and enthusiasm, as well as loss of ability to concentrate, to remember, to think clearly, along with the loss of bodily functions like sleep, appetite, weight control and bowel movement. Characteristically, the sufferer of depression has difficulty in sleeping, wakes in the early hours, and experiences a loss of weight. Depression as an illness can occur in man, woman or child, and it is to be differentiated from depression as an emotion of sadness, such as occurs to us all when we hear of a tragic happening. On the other hand, the depression which occurs in premenstrual syndrome and postnatal depression is a hormonal depression and differs from the typical depressive illness in that:

1. the timing is shorter and predictable;
2. its duration can be measured in days, rather than the weeks, months or years of depressive illness;
3. it is characterised by weight gain and increased appetite, cravings and binges in contrast to the weight loss and diminishing appetite in typical depression;
4. there is a yearning for sleep, and women tend to stay in bed all day, differentiating them from those with typical depression who are awake in the early hours and cannot stay in bed but get up and make tea or even do the housework;
5. distinctively marked irritability and sudden changes of mood accompany the premenstrual depression.

The depression of premenstrual syndrome also differs from manic depression in its timing. Whereas in manic depressions the state of depression following the manic state usually lasts for many weeks or months and is quite unpredictable, depression of premenstrual syndrome never lasts more than 14 days and usually is even less, moreover they are predictable in the time of their return. In premenstrual syndrome, the elated and excited state of mania which sometimes occurs is intimately associated with the depression which occurs as a rapid mood change, often on the same day.

Table 8.1 Characteristics of Premenstrual Syndrome Depression

1.	Shorter, limited to 14 days at longest
2.	Predictable recurrence each premenstruum
3.	Increased appetite with food cravings and binges
4.	Weight gain
5.	Yearning for sleep
6.	Marked irritability

As long ago as 1855, Marce, the French physician, observed that when puerperal psychosis or postnatal depression improves, the symptoms ease after menstruation, only to return again before the next menstruation. There is then a gradual transition over the months with greater improvement of symptoms in the postmenstruum, but with recurrences in the premenstruum. Gradually as symptoms disappear in the postmenstruum a stage of premenstrual syndrome is reached with symptoms limited only to the premenstruum (Dalton 1989) (Figure 8.1).

It is suggested that postnatal depression results from the difficulty experienced by some women in adjusting to the abrupt drop in progesterone level which occurs at delivery (Figure 4.3) (Dalton, 1971). Postnatal depression may be

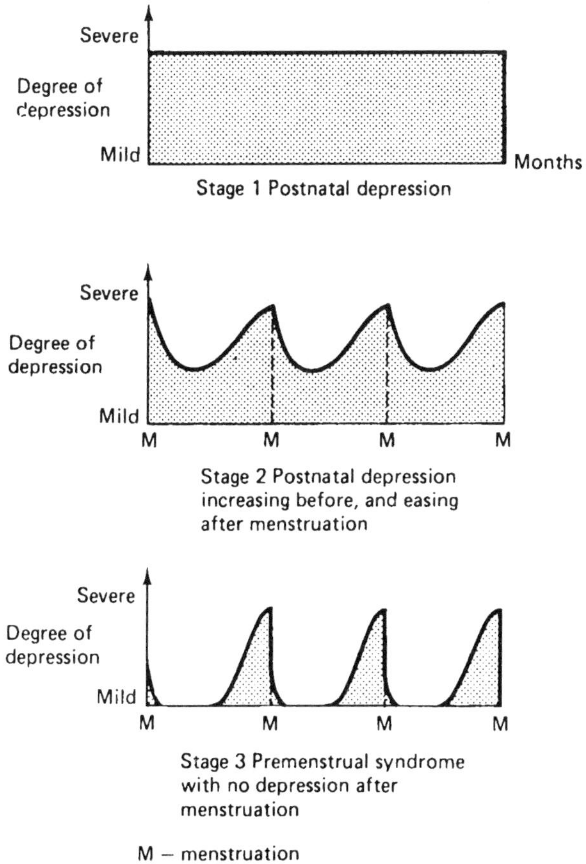

Figure 8.1 Stages as postnatal depression changes to premenstrual syndrome. *From Dalton K. (1989). Depression After Childbirth, Oxford University Press, 2nd Edition.*

prevented by the administration of progesterone immediately on completion of labour and continued for the next two months or until the first menstruation occurs after child birth (Dalton 1985, 1989 and 1990). Premenstrual depression is associated with a feeling of uselessness, loneliness, endless crying, of being unloved and not worthy of affection and is followed by feelings of guilt. One repeatedly hears such statements as, 'I spend hours in the loo where no-one can touch me'... 'I lie in bed all day'... 'I run off to the barn'... 'who cares'... 'I don't deserve to be here'... 'No-one else is as ugly... look at me'... 'There's a devil within me... it's ticking away... it'll erupt like a volcano'.

> P.W. wrote, 'The black cloud descends ten days before my period and drives me to drink. So far I've abused dozens of people, I tried to kill myself by crashing the car, setting fire to the house, and attacking my husband verbally and physically until he retaliated and put me in hospital. This led to a divorce, another breakdown, then a reconciliation. I become so depressed, something takes me over and I become demented. This month I've gone through hell and today, the first day of bleeding, I feel I have come out of the depths of my private hell and am glad to be here – but for how much longer can I cope'.

> A.C. wrote, 'Two weeks before my period is due I seem to be completely irrational. My emotions become monsters. I buy stupid clothes, become very dissatisfied. Then I begin feeling fear, I want to see no-one. I want to hide. I feel ugly inside and out, everything goes wrong, I have no mental or physical energy. Again, I get a raging compulsion to hurt myself or kill myself. Thus far I have been able to hang on to the very small sane voice inside me, but last month I injured myself, though not badly, and punched the wall. When my period starts, these awful feelings lift. I then have a good week. Oh, it is good, good to be alive, to be positive, to do. I make plans, get things started, they are discarded with resignation a week later.'

During the days of depression all insight is lost, there is no hope or prospect of improvement, and with this feeling that there is no tomorrow and no one cares, the scope for wrongdoing is wide open. A woman in Arizona, where the temperature is perpetually above 75°, bought herself a full length mink coat, 'I didn't care...no-one else cares...I wanted to love myself'. She's still paying for it three years later. Another woman when in this state of mind, bought three new cars in one day. This is the time that some women shoplift clothes, dresses, jewellery and perfume. Is it to comfort themselves? Nobody knows, for their minds are irrational. A taxi driver described how his wife would steal gold watches each month, and he would dutifully return them to the understanding shopkeeper. Some women describe the difficulty of returning the stolen articles a few days later. They don't want the item, they don't like the item and they are terrified of being caught with it.

> J.T., 43 years old nurse, was charged with shoplifting. Her husband had recognised her premenstrual confusion and absentmindedness for four years since the birth of their third child. She would prepare lists before going shopping but she would still come home with the wrong items, food the children could not eat and girls clothes for her sons. She would forget to collect the children from school, put cabbage to cook in the washing up machine and make porridge out of tea bags and milk. At work they teased her that she suffered from Alzheimers disease. On the day of the incident she was returning some shoes and a skirt which she had bought but were quite the wrong size. She left her car in a car park but couldn't remember which one, and the police had to mount a search for it. Until this brush with the law her husband had not been unduly worried by his wife's premenstrual quirks as he knew when to expect them.

❑ Suicide

When depression is at its deepest, suicide attempts either successful or unsuccessful, may be made. The attempt may be by swallowing an excessive number of tablets, jumping from a height or running in front of a car or train. Surveys as far apart as London, Los Angeles and Delhi have confirmed that half of all female suicides occur during the paramenstruum (MacKinnon and MacKinnon 1956, Gregory 1957, Dalton

1989, Riberio 1962, Mandell & Mandell 1967, Wetzel and McClure 1972). Although women make more attempts at suicide than men, the men succeed more frequently until the age of 50 years when this masculine success rate disappears. Dr. John Pollitt, speaking at the Royal Society of Medicine in 1976, suggested that:

> "Perhaps one reason for the female's lack of success is that the majority of attempts are made during the premenstruum or menstruation. Killing oneself is not easy: success requires careful planning. Women in the premenstrual phase show a marked tendency to be careless, thoughtless, unpunctual, forgetful and absentminded. This inefficiency at a time when they are more likely to try and end their lives may result in a disproportionate number of failures".

Whilst one appreciates that a suicide gesture represents a cry for help, an attention seeking gesture and a need for love and attention, one must not forget the other cries for help such as slashing the wrist, arson and hoax telephone calls, these are dealt with in Chapter 10.

❑ Irritability

Sudden mood changes with unexpected irritability and fury at a chance remark or minimal provocation are frequent among premenstrual syndrome sufferers during the premenstruum. In the mild case it may result merely in a sarcastic remark or be the end of conversation, but in the severe examples the woman may become irrational, illogical, impatient, hostile, aggressive and violent. She may suddenly shout or scream, slam the table and bang doors, throw knives, plates, books, ashtrays and smash windows or doors, and assault her husband, children, teachers, police or neighbours. At the end of such a hysterical outburst, there may be copious crying, or she may run away and lock herself in her bedroom or drive in a fury down the motorway. In one case the couple were evicted from their hotel at 2 a.m. Another woman, after throwing the furniture out of the second floor window, jumped out herself ending up in hospital with multiple bruises.

Sudden episodic loss of self control or loss of temper following slight provocation, is sometimes called the 'dyscontrol syndrome' ('dys' meaning 'bad' 'difficult' or 'abnormal'), and this can occur in men or women. In premenstrual syndrome, the sudden loss of control is especially liable to occur when the woman has had a long interval without eating some complex carbohydrate, such as may occur when the husband comes home in the evening and the wife has not eaten, or barely eaten, all day (see Chapters 12 and 13).

> On 11th April, 1981 J. B. wrote: ' I tried to lock myself in the bedroom away from the children until my husband came but I was drawn downstairs by Sarah screaming. She couldn't get to the toilet as Kim (20 months) was sitting behind the gate at the top of the stairs. She was panicking, and as I pushed Keith away to get her down, he fell backwards down the stairs and cut his top lip and bruised his head. Immediately I rang my husband as his mouth was bleeding. The Social Services called, I took Kim to the doctor. Later that evening they called with a Court Order and both children were placed in a place of safety for 28 days. Last month when I was having a particularly irritable day, Kim broke a toy in front of me. I beat him and bruised him. Kim was placed on the Child Abuse Register. I just cannot understand why this happens to me every time I start menstruation.'

> An extract from D. F.'s medical report reads: 'The evening prior to admission she had a row with her husband and the next day grabbed a customer and blamed her for the demise of the shop, and threw the customer out of the door. She then became aggressive and confused, and her husband called the police.'

❑ Psychosis

Psychosis is grossly abnormal behaviour which may present as confusion, delusions, hallucinations or paranoia (persecution mania). She may be confused and troubled by ruminative and disturbing thoughts. She may complain of feelings of unreality, 'like living in a bubble', or 'things go strange, everything hates me'.

> M.D. a 24 year old secretary explained: 'The feeling in my

> head alternated with headache, which moved, to complete the confusion. The most frightening aspect was the sensation of my mouth, which I felt was leaving my face and going over to the wall. It was outside my control to do anything, so I tried to remain calm and go about as normal'.

A woman's strange actions, such as searching for cakes in the wardrobe or exclaiming 'I've lost my foot', may alert others to the onset of the delusions. She may be observed walking along the street talking to herself, suddenly stopping as if she sees or hears something strange. She may give totally inappropriate answers. She may be confused with relationships, believing that her brother is really her father, or falsely recalling her past life in India, when in reality she has never moved more than 5 miles from her Essex village. She may still, each premenstruum, not be able to forgive herself for the mistakes she made at school twenty years ago.

The hallucinations may be either visual, when she sees something or somebody, or auditory, when she hears somebody. They may be compulsive, issuing non-stop instructions which must be obeyed, regardless of how absurd or dangerous the action may be. Often the visual hallucinations are frightening and grotesque.

With the onset of temporary psychosis, it often remains a matter of chance whether the woman is admitted to a mental hospital or charged with a crime. If she is still confused and deluded at the time she is apprehended, she is more likely to be admitted to hospital. On the other hand if she is completely normal and fully recovered when the offence is discovered the chances are that she will be prosecuted.

> A 45 year old housewife from Hertfordshire was charged with shoplifting. She was asked to accompany the plain-clothes police officer to the police station. On the journey she noticed that he had brown socks and black shoes and was proceeding along the same Dunstable Road that a rapist had once used. She accused the police officer of being a rapist having the same clothes and using the same route. On arrival at the police station the officer 'phoned the local mental hospital to see if anyone of her description was missing. Her husband and elder daugh-

ter confirmed that the defendant had these strange episodes each premenstruum, but they did not know that treatment was available. The case was dismissed and progesterone therapy started, which removed her periodic cyclical episodes of confusion.

A 15 year old Michigan schoolgirl imagined she was the Great Goddess, so vitally important to the world that she could walk across the road and all traffic would stop. She could go into a shop, buy to her heart's content and that her invisible body guard would pay. On each occasion she was hospitalised and within two days menstruation would start. On other occasions she tore down the drapes and walked on the furniture. She received 'messages from God and demons in her room'. She dressed inappropriately with strange hairdos and was sexually aggressive. After seven short hospitalisations her parents realised that the episodes always occurred premenstrually, were shortlived and ended by the second day of menstruation. Following transatlantic 'phone calls, progesterone treatment was organised with her psychiatrist and gynaecologist. When seen six months later and again after two years there had been no further episodes, she has graduated from college, and succeeded in gradually reducing progesterone.

The 14 year old daughter of an education officer in Indiana had short lived episodes of psychosis. She had strange ideation, received messages from magazines, believed trucks were watching her home, kicked a hole in the living room wall, got confused and went to the wrong apartment, had angry outbursts and was out of touch with reality. Following her four hospitalisations in which she had been diagnosed as 'adolescent anxiety', 'paranoid', 'atypical psychosis' and 'bi-polar manic depression', her parents recognised the occurrence was always in the premenstruum. On one occasion she started to menstruate when in the admission ward. The parents knew that the brainstorm would soon subside, so they waited a few hours and then took her home without treatment or admission. The next day at breakfast she asked innocently 'When are you going to have the door and window mended? How did it get broken?'. She had complete amnesia of the incident. Again following a, series of transatlantic 'phone calls, progesterone therapy was started and the girl has had no further incidents in the last five years.

Another problem is the recurrence of ideas of persecution which may recur premenstrually.

The 40 year old mother who had one son, discovered her husband had a brief extramarital affair. The wife was reasonably upset initially, but over the months she gradually forgave him. However, after two years when she restarted using the contraceptive pill she developed paranoid ideas regarding the affair. She would taunt her husband, question him, watch him and accuse him of infidelity. One night for no obvious reason she started to grill her husband about the possibility that he was paying for the flat occupied by the lady to whom he had once made an overture. She continued to harangue until eventually he lost his temper and smacked her face. She admitted to having these crazy thoughts in her head which she could not control, they would only last a day or two and then recede until the next premenstruum. When progesterone treatment was started marital harmony was restored.

Endo and his colleagues (1978) reported menstrually related psychosis in seven girls aged between 13 and 25 years, in which there was manic-confusion, retardation, auditory and visual hallucinations, delusions and paranoia and they cite other examples in Japanese medical literature.

❑ Husband's reaction

How does or how should a husband react to such monthly irritability? He may either remain silent, leave the room, go to sleep, or he may try to justify himself. If he answers, she shouts louder. If he tries to calm her, she will become even more abusive. If sooner or later he assaults her, she will become the battered wife. Or he might separate, although his love for her will persist for the rest of the month, or will he find another woman who is less volatile?

There is a high incidence of divorce among sufferers of premenstrual syndrome, although the actual rate is difficult to determine in a society where so many couples are living together. If a relationship breaks up should that be considered a divorce? How long must a couple have been together before she becomes a common law wife? Clare's (1983) study demonstrated a statistically significant and positive relationship between disturbances in marital function and premenstrual complainers which was independent of psychiatric status.

❑ Nymphomania

Nymphomania, which was noticed by Pritchard one hundred and fifty years ago is still a problem today. Israel (1938), Gray (1941) and Hart (1960) have confirmed its recurrence in the premenstruum. Although increased libido is present in adolescents and childless women, there is more likely to be loss of libido after child birth particularly if the pregnancy was followed by postnatal depression. This increase in libido premenstrually differentiates it from depressive illness in which a loss of libido lasts throughout the month.

The headmistress of a girls' approved school in North England described how the girls would escape once a month during their premenstruum, only to be found in the local cafes where the boys congregated.

> A sixteen year old schoolgirl would periodically abscond from home, sometimes in her nightgown, giving as her reasons "I'm Adam's wife, I have a duty to procreate the world ", "God told me to go out...You don't believe God or me "... "Hitler didn't kill himself... I know... I'm his wife... I must find him".

❑ Alcohol and drug abuse

Many women have urges for alcohol which are limited to the premenstruum at which time they become quickly intoxicated with no more than their usual amount of alcohol. They then are able to abstain without much difficulty in the postmenstruum. The alcoholic agencies refer to such women as once-a-month-ers, differentiating them from men who tend to be chronic alcoholics requiring daily replenishment. The problem in the premenstruum is probably related to slower detoxification of alcohol by the liver. This tends to be increased when there is also a problem of fluid retention.

Belfer and Carroll (1971) noted that 67% of menstruating female alcoholics related their drinking bouts to the paramenstruum, and 100% indicated that drinking had begun or increased in the premenstruum. Unfortunately, those women with premenstrual depression have a propensity to take to alcohol to relieve their depression.

Similarly, there is a tendency to abuse drugs premenstrually, especially the tranquillisers prescribed to ease the premenstrual irritability and tension. There is then a great temptation to take more to increase the effect. Overdose of drugs is the commonest method of attempted suicide in the premenstruum, because drugs are so easily obtainable.

> S.W., 34 year old state registered nurse, was an alcoholic, with numerous mental hospital admissions. One day it was recognised by a staff nurse that the alcoholic episodes only occurred premenstrually. The staff nurse accompanied her on her first clinic visit to ensure that the full extent of her problems were appreciated and that the correct treatment would be carried out. Progesterone therapy was successful in transforming her life, and she started working again. After three years she lapsed, and she wrote:
>
> "About ten days ago I began not sleeping, feeling slightly depressed and possibly lethargic. Fearing it might be the old problem, I immediately returned to progesterone suppositories but too late. I went to my doctor and obtained 60 Dalmane 15 mg tablets. For a couple of nights I took as prescribed, but then I abused them with alcohol (the old story!). The next 5-6 days are virtually a blank. I assaulted a policewoman and have to appear in court. I remember spending one night in a foul police cell shivering like an animal and trying to strangle myself with my tights. One or two nights spent either in local mental hospital or general one. I was going to be sectioned (29), but the consultant said "I can find nothing mentally wrong with this girl to detain her". As you know

at the moment I am doing a post-graduate course at Liverpool University and appear to be coping very well".

This chapter has presented on overall view of symptoms which cause criminal actions. The examples presented are a small selection from the records of the many patients who have been helped back to a normal life. They have been carefully selected to give a good picture of the infinite variety of manifestations to which the practitioner must be alerted in his search for evidence, all the while keeping in mind the precise time relationship of the event. It is important to realise that only some of the patients described here ended up in court, many were settled out of court. Fortunately there were enough people aware of the diagnosis of premenstrual syndrome to ensure that treatment was started for these sick people before they were branded with the stigma of being a criminal.

Chapters 9 and 10 will be dealing specifically with 'violence' and 'cries for help'.

❑ References

Belfer M.L. & Carroll M. (1971). *Arch. Gen. Psychiat.;* **25**, 540.
Clare A.W. (1983). *'Psychiatric and Social Aspects of Pre Menstrual Complainers';* Psychol: Med: Supp; **4**.
Dalton K. (1960). *Brit. Med. J.;* **2**, 1647–1649.
Dalton K. (1961). *Brit. Med. J.;* **2**, 1752–1753.
Dalton K. (1971). *Proc. Roy. Soc. Med.;* **64**, 12, 1249-1252.
Dalton K. (1984). *Premenstrual Syndrome and Progesterone Therapy*, William Heinemann Medical Books, London & Year Book Medical Publishers Inc., Chicago.
Dalton K. (1985). *Practitioner;* **229**, 507–8.
Dalton K. (1989). *Depression after Childbirth;* 2nd edition, Oxford University Press, Oxford.
Dalton K. (1989). *Int: J. Prenatal and Perinatal Studies;* 323-327
D'Orban P.T. & Dalton J. (1980). *Psycholog. Med.;* **10**, 35–359.
Endo M., Daiguji M., Asana Y., Yamashita I & Takahashi S. (1978). *J. Clin. Psychiat.;* 456–466.
Gray L.A. (1941). *Sth. Med. J.;* **34**, 1004.
Grefory B.A. (1957). *J. Psychosom. Res.;* **2**, 61.

Hart R.D. (1960). *Brit, Med. J.;* **1**, 1023.
Israel S.L. (1938). *J. Amer. Med. Ass.;* **110**, 1721.
MacKinnon P.C.B. & MacKinnon I.L. (1956). *Brit. Med. J.;* 555
Pollitt J. (1977). *Proc. Roy. Soc. Med.;* **70**, 145.
Ribeiro A.L. (1962). *Brit. Med. J.;* **1**, 590.
Wetzel R.D. & McClure J.N. (1972). *Comprehensive Psych.;* **13**, 4, 369.

9

Violence

Violence is at the extreme end of a range of irritabilities that progress from an irrational emotional involvement until they erupt in an outbreak of violence, either verbal or physical. It appears to commence with a smouldering resentment, progresses to anger, which becomes seething, and on into a cantankerous and irrational hostility before exploding in violence. Once started along the emotional path, it becomes almost impossible to avoid.

The British Medical Journal periodically invites a leading authority to answer a question dealing with his or her speciality.

In 1984 Ian Oswald, Professor of psychiatry at Edinburgh was invited to answer the question "What is meant by the term 'explosive temperament' and is it treatable?" He replied:

> 'Explosive temperament is merely a descriptive term for someone who has a bad temper, who does not control it, and whose outbursts are out of all proportion to the circumstances'.

The Professor's answer seems to be that of a rational mind searching for a rational explanation of the irrational event of an irrational mind, for later in his reply he states that nothing can be done, but that one must wait – 'as they slowly mature to a more mellow middle age'. He is referring to a medical condition which defies treatment.

Many of those contained in our special hospitals come into the category of having explosive temperaments, but it is well to recall that 90% of convicted criminals are men. In women there is a category of explosive violence with an identifiable cause which responds admirably to the correct treatment.

The violence of premenstrual syndrome is predictable in its time of occurrence and is most certainly hormonal in its derivation. It occurs in the premenstruum and disappears with the onset of menstruation, this is the hallmark of premenstrual syndrome. The precise day of its occurrence within those 14 premenstrual days is not so predictable. The husband will awake one morning and sense immediately that this is going to be one of those days. If he brings her a cup of tea or coffee it might be thrown over him or be knocked to the floor. He knows that nothing he does will be right. He desperately wants to comfort and help his wife, but knows from experience that whatever he does, he cannot escape the inevitable explosion, for it is veritably a programmed time bomb and there is no means of defusing it.

Meanwhile, the woman herself may also have awakened sensing that it is going to be that sort of day. However strong willed she may have been yesterday, that strength has evaporated overnight and she is powerless to think coherently or act rationally or consciously. Indeed, the very comfort and love her body may yearn for is physically rejected by a mind that seems to have gone haywire. She has no insight into her condition or her actions and any awareness she may have left is only that once menstruation starts this bad dream will go away. It is in this nightmare state that violence can erupt and endow the woman with phenomenal physical strength, although she has no idea of what damage she may be doing with it. It is the irresistible impulse that directs the action. In such a situation there can be no *'mens rea'* or guilty intent.

It is the young women under 25 years, who are often the most violent.They are the ones ready to attack teachers, boyfriends, parents and young children at the slightest provocation or for no apparent reason. They may be judged to have a sadistic streak, but there is no knowing what went on in their mind immediately before the killing or outburst. What irrational, uncontrolled, compulsive thought compelled her action? The other group at risk of violence are those acting under the influence of alcohol or drugs, and this group includes both the young women and the depressed, middle aged housewives. D'Orban and Dalton (1980) investigated fifty women being held in custody and charged with crimes of violence, of whom 64% had committed violence against the person and 86% against property. They found 44% of the violent crimes had been committed in the paramenstruum (P=<0.02).

Within a few days of entering practice I recall one evening

being visited by a couple, both holding a blood stained towel to their faces. He had a laceration on his forehead requiring four sutures, and she had two nasty cuts on her scalp, which also received four sutures, just to be fair. The next week the wife came in alone to have the sutures removed . 'I'm terribly sorry I lied to you last week – I always tell the truth'. Not being able to recall the incident she was asked to explain, 'Doc, when we two bloody messes came in, you asked, 'What have you been up to?'. We said the kitchen shelf had fallen down and hit us. But it wasn't that Doc . – we only had our usual flaming row I threw a tin opener at him. I always tell the truth.' She had been in her premenstruum at the time of her fight. So she unexpectedly received instructions on how to record such events on a menstrual chart, which later gave a positive diagnosis of premenstrual syndrome. Their marriage was much happier once hormone therapy was started.

It is such incidents that remind one of the milder forms of violence, like hitting and smashing, which are such common happenings in the privacy of the home but which only rarely appear in public.

V.W. wrote asking for help. 'I have been married for 24 years and we have seven children between 22 years and 7 years. I have never, until the last few years, done anything about my PMS, although it has caused terrible scenes and fights as I seem to go crazy and become very, very violent. I have several times tried to kill my husband by strangling him, often waking in the night, and in my mind would be the thought that he was hurting me and I would attack him. This may not make much sense to you as it is difficult to remember, as when I woke in the morning I would only remember that he hit me. It seemed as if I just hated him as a different person for maybe a week or ten days every month. Over the years he tried to help me in various ways, talking, hitting me back, or first holding me down, but I would never really explain it to my doctor as I thought he would think me crazy'.

P.G. was an attractive blonde with pink and white complexion, spoilt by a 2 inch recent scar on her left cheek.

> She was accompanied by her fiance, also with a healing scar on his face, apparently the result of an argument involving a flower vase. He was anxious to be sure that his fiancee fully explained the problems of her monthly outbursts of temper. He had kept a useful chart, which confirmed that the explosions occurred in relation to menstruation. She was started on progesterone therapy. The next visit six weeks later, again revealed that both had facial bruising, the result of a fight somehow involving an attache case. Obviously the dose of progesterone was insufficient so it was doubled. The third visit two months later was all smiles. They were going to get married after all, her tantrums had disappeared and they brought an attache case as a thank you gift.

It was an inconspicuous item in a London evening newspaper in October, 1964, which first drew my attention to the effect of mother's menstruation on her child.

> The item told of a young mother who had beaten up her 3 year old daughter. In evidence the mother stated 'I suffer from my nerves, at certain times of the month it is worse than others'. The husband said 'She seems quite uncontrollable. I have restrained my wife physically'.

This young woman reminded me of a similar instance in which one of my kind and motherly patients, in a fit of temper, had struck her child, fracturing the fibula. In her case these violent outbursts always occurred just before menstruation, and treatment for her premenstrual tension resulted in a happy and even-tempered mother (Dalton 1966).

A child wants love and knows when he's rejected. If he accidentally breaks a toy or makes a mess he doesn't want to be spanked and doesn't understand why some days mother is so much stricter than other days. To some it seems that premenstrual syndrome is the commonest cause of non-accidental injury. In 1970 the National Society for the Prevention of Cruelty to Children were planning a survey into battered babies at which I spoke about premenstrual baby battering and also talked to the social workers who were going to participate in the project. It was agreed that when the social workers called to investigate, a few questions should be asked about the date of the last menstruation. After an interval of some months, enquiries revealed that the three questions relating to menstruation were considered too personal to be asked at the first visit, and therefore the questions would be delayed for a few months before discussing so delicate a subject, but with such a delay the answers would have no relevance. That was 20 years ago, so in short it was completely neglected. Five years ago I received a letter from an Inspector of the NSPCC who wrote spontaneously to me stating:

> 'At the present time child abuse that is caused by premenstrual syndrome is obscured by prejudice and disinterest. Premenstrual syndrome is perceived as a serious problem, which is neglected by everyone other than the women who study or suffer it'.

The NSPCC must see more violence inflicted on children as a consequence of premenstrual syndrome than any other organisation, yet at present they remain blind to it.

The problem of the care of children who have been abused during bouts of premenstrual violence is different from that of those whose mothers abuse at random. Once a positive diagnosis of premenstrual syndrome has been made and treatment started, then the children can remain with their parents reasonably safely, subject to sensible precautions. Women suffering from premenstrual syndrome are usually motherly types, who love their children, and once treated they give the necessary physical and emotional support to the developing children. Therefore, every effort should be made to ensure that the children are not taken into public care in such cases.

> Even before a positive diagnosis of premenstrual syndrome was made, C.R. would drop the children in on friends before stopping at the corner shop to buy two bottles of vodka, which she would then consume alone in the peace of her home.
>
> Mrs. L.A., whose premenstrual irritability often ended in child abuse, arranged for her mother to stay with her for the one vulnerable week each month to care for the three children.
>
> Mrs. J.B. a paramedical, had abused her two children who were removed from her care and taken to her mother. Six months later, when she moved away, the order was

revoked as Mrs. B. then knew and understood the problem and made arrangements to take the children to a named friend nearby whenever she had any early premenstrual symptoms. That was three years ago, and apart from social meetings aimed at familiarisation for the children, there has been no need for emergency care, but the knowledge that a bolthole is available is very helpful.

Severe premenstrual syndrome can occur equally in all social classes and at all levels of intelligence. However, when premenstrual violence occurs in the mentally handicapped woman, who would not in any case be expected to explain her uncontrollable impulse, she is regarded as a disturbed mentally handicapped woman. Nevertheless, with the disturbed mentally handicapped it is still useful and may be important to note carefully the days of unprovoked violence. If there is a correlation between disturbed behaviour and menstruation then progesterone treatment is of value, although it will not overcome the mental handicap.

E.R., 34 years old, was in a home for mentally disturbed adults. She was observed making assaults in relation to menstruation which stopped with progesterone treatment.

A.U., 20 years old, also mentally handicapped and with occasional outbursts, attended a day centre where she might suddenly throw an iron or other item across the room or would suddenly attack or bite the individual sitting next to her at meals. She, too, responded to progesterone treatment and the violent outbursts ended.

A.B. was regarded as of normal ability until puberty, when disturbed behaviour started and was noted to be related to menstruation. She was given the pill for fifteen years as well as tranquillisers and antidepressants. When seen at the age of 37 years, because of menstrual violence, the pill was stopped, progesterone treatment started and the dose gradually increased while stopping her other medication. Her whole personality changed, she resumed her education and succeeded in passing three 'A' levels (the advanced grade of school leaving certificate), she has improved her grades and is now hoping to enter university.

M. J. was first seen in 1970 with premenstrual epilepsy, so severe that her two children, 6 and 4 years old, were taken into care. On progesterone treatment the premenstrual epilepsy disappeared and the children were returned to her, and her driving licence restored. She started training as a mental health nurse, won all the prizes during her training, and after 12 years became the warden in charge of a hostel for disturbed mentally handicapped women. She is an excellent diagnostician of premenstrual syndrome among the inmates under her care. She has a thorough understanding of the disease and has helped innumerable women.

The best self help measures for those with aggressive tendencies are energetic sports like tennis, squash or golf, where the aim is to hit even harder and harder, to stretch to the limit, to use up all the extra adrenalin and then relax with a glow of exhaustion. Unfortunately this outlet is thoroughly impractical for sufferers from premenstrual syndrome, in whom the premenstruum is accompanied by lethargy, a feeling of 'far too much to do', and an overwhelming desire to put off until tomorrow all good resolutions.

A schoolfriend hoped she'd be rich enough one day to allot one room strictly for the throwing of books and bottles of ink. Books make such a lovely flutter if thrown properly, and only a small amount of ink makes a frightful mess.

This chapter makes a frightening, gloomy picture of a violent society, but that is not so, for we must remember that premenstrual violence only occurs in less than 1% of the female population of menstruating age. Furthermore, once it has been correctly diagnosed as premenstrual syndrome and properly treated with prophylactic progesterone, the whole problem disappears.

❑ References

Dalton K. (1966). *Proc. Roy. Soc. Med.;* **59**, 10, 1014–1016.
D'Orban P.T. and Dalton J. (1980). *Psycholog. Med.;* **10**, 353–359.
Oswald I. (1984). *Brit. Med. J.;* **288**, 1511.

10

'SOS – Cry for Help'

In the Morse code, 'SOS' is an internationally recognised cry for help which was used by all ships on the high seas in the days of wireless telegraphy to call for assistance. In these days of radio communication, the words 'MAYDAY, MAYDAY' alert all who hear them to a distress call whether on land, sea or in the air, and when heard the call is always acknowledged and assistance races to the scene.

What a pity no one has thought of a similar brief international call sign for those poor distressed women who are at the end of their tether and try to alert help by various bizarre actions. Several relief and help organisations including Samaritans and NAPS, (the National Association for Premenstrual Syndrome) have set up crisis lines on the telephone, but this is no help if the distressed woman has no telephone to use or is too confused to remember the number and fumbles her dialling. Only a few of the grotesque actions they resort to contain any criminal or civil intent, but they all involve either police, fire or medical services to a greater or lesser extent. Significantly many of these women are suffering from undiagnosed premenstrual syndrome which could be properly treated.

With the mind in a jumble and sinking inevitably deeper into the pit of despair, where can one turn for help? In the dazed state, all alone, how can one make the agonies and miseries understood? Is it not best to end it all? There are those who try to end it all, some successfully, but most unsuccessfully, particularly for those in the shortlived muddled premenstrual depression. Once drastic steps have been taken however, society wakes up. It has heard the cri de coeur, and efforts are made to provide love, help and sympathy to overcome the loneliness of mind and body. Although suicide is no longer a crime in law, it still remains to many a moral evil.

> One women wrote, 'I have for ever the guilt of one who has tried to take her own life'.

Suicide attempts are a sign of pathological depression or a muddled mind demanding urgent attention. But apart from suicide, other ways of alerting society are sometimes used, such as wrist slashing, arson and hoax telephone calls. Society's aim should be to spot those who are desperate before such drastic measures are taken and to let them know that help is at hand. Here the Samaritans deserve a special bouquet for they do marvellous work. Doctors are ready and able to help the fight back to normality, particularly when the problem is recurrent, but shortlived, as in premenstrual syndrome. It is the very recurrence of depression that makes premenstrual syndrome so appalling, as one expressed it:

> 'In the good normal days I wake up happy and ready to face the day, but all the time dreading the return of the inevitable low, hoping that next month there will be the strength to fight the horrors – but that's impossible, there's no insight when at the bottom of the pit'.
>
> L. L. now a 30 year old secretary, recalled 'At school, seeing some ropes in the drying room I contemplated hanging myself. Another time on a family holiday in Wales, I tried to strangle myself. Somehow someone understood and helped me.'

Some premenstrual suicide attempts are totally inadequate, and these women are easier to re-establish back to normal life with hormone treatment. Some are successful, however, leaving behind a trail of sorrow, a broken hearted widower who must face life alone with the guilt for having let it happen and for having failed to be alert to his wife's predicament. There may also be children, now motherless, who face a struggle in a one parent family. Others fail only partially, and theirs is the most tragic predicament. A young girl jumped in front of an underground train and severed her right arm. The surgeons fought throughout the night to repair every nerve and blood vessel microscopically, but two years later, after a further ten operations, she is still left with a useless, paralysed right arm, inadequate for the task of coping with two young children. The housewife whose aspirin overdose damaged her kidneys which now will never recover fully from the onslaught. These are among the real tragedies and all were preventable if the depth of the recurrent premenstrual depression in these women had been recognised earlier.

The irresistible impulse that suddenly forces a woman to slash her wrist with some broken glass, a razor blade or penknife, must be seen as an attention seeking episode or a cry of desperation. This is particularly common in young teenagers in whom the cry must be taken seriously even if the wound is only skin deep. Incidentally, Table 3.3 showed that these instances of self mutilation were characteristic of the premenstrual syndrome offenders. In every case, the slashing preceded the criminal offence by months or years and was associated with premenstrual syndrome, which suggests that the whole declining personality and lifestyle could have been halted at an earlier stage. Another reminder for us to consider the possible diagnosis of premenstrual syndrome in the young pubertal girl.

Some women who injure themselves severely appear to be completely anaesthetised and feel no pain during the process. Could that be the surge of endorphins, the body's opiates, that Reid and Yen (1981) implicate in the etiology of premenstrual syndrome? One woman wielded an axe to her head doing irreparable damage. However not all women are so anaesthetised during their cry for help.

> Carol described in a T.V. interview in, 'Pull yourself Together, Woman', how she was wrapped in a towel when attempting to cut her wrists, as she didn't want to see what she was doing to herself. In the end her attempt failed, and she ran into the street for help.

The healing of scars differs depending on many factors, including the site of injury. Some lacerations on the face open up quickly and always require suturing to prevent an ugly scar. Others, for no known reason, overheal and end up with hard, red, raised, disfiguring keloid scars. After treatment for premenstrual syndrome, when a new lifestyle has been developed, such disfiguring scars can be removed by cosmetic surgery, but there's no guarantee that the next scar will be perfect.

> L.B. is now 29 years old, well adjusted and leading a very full life. She was threatened with expulsion from school at 14 years, but her mother, who had previously benefited from progesterone treatment, recognised the

monthly displays of temper tantrums and antisocial behaviour and arranged for progesterone treatment, which L.B. still requires. She recalled recently how, as part of her sixth form studies, she attended court and on another occasion the police station. It was there, in company with the other sixth formers, that she saw a beautiful brunette brought in, who had smashed a window to obtain some glass to slash her wrist. This had a marked effect on the schoolgirls, who appeared to appreciate the tragedy of the situation and the depth of despair that had driven the woman to the act. But they could not understand why she should now have a criminal record, when all she needed was medical treatment. Why is it that the sixth formers could recognise a sick mind when society at large would prefer to punish?

The women, whose premenstrual depression reaches a stage where, in a cry for help, they make a hoax 'phone call pose a problem. They are a nuisance to the emergency services for they cannot be ignored. Full action is required on every occasion, and if it's a bomb hoax, the members of the public are also inconvenienced as streets, shops and offices are vacated.

Police spent more than 350 hours following up bogus clues to a teenager's murder after 'phone calls from a woman claiming to know the killer. Mrs. S. N., 29 year old mother of two hyperactive children, told the court she "desperately wanted to talk to someone". She was put on probation for wasting police time.

A 19 year old, unemployed childless woman, had her first menstruation at 16 years and the next year began to display criminal behaviour at monthly intervals, usually making false emergency calls, for which she was initially given probation, later Borstal training and then prison sentences. However, her offences continued even during detention. Offences occurred during the last two premenstrual days and the first two days of menstruation. She said that on her premenstrual days she was irritable, depressed, violent and felt like 'walking out of life'. She claimed she had often asked for help in the premenstruum when she felt a sudden urge to jump out of a window or assault someone. This was confirmed by a prison officer's statement, 'Feels she will smash up. Doesn't want to leave prison', and a report from Borstal, which said 'she sometimes asked to be put in a cell alone as she felt safe there', (Dalton 1980). She received progesterone treatment with benefit in prison, but unfortunately on her release from prison her injections were not resumed for seven days during which she committed another hoax 'phone offence. She was taken into custody, but three weeks later she alerted the staff at the hostel that she felt violent. The next day before injections could be obtained, she threw a knife at a man, escaped from the hostel, made another hoax emergency call and assaulted three policemen. She started to menstruate that night in the prison. That was 6 years ago, on progesterone therapy she is well, happily married and currently pregnant.

If only all these women could be implanted with electronic bleepers triggered by their hormones as their critical time approaches, they might alert all within range to their hormonal cry for help.

❑ References

Dalton K. (1980). *Lancet 2*, 1070-1071.
Reid R L. & Yen SSC (1980). *Amer J. Ostet Gynaecol;* **139**, 25-102.

11

Finding the Evidence

The normal rules of evidence apply, all evidence must be factual and not hearsay. Material evidence produced must be pure fact, and witnesses called to confirm the defendant's statements must also produce factual evidence and not conjectural evidence. It is of no value to state repeatedly 'but it always happens before menstruation'. If using premenstrual syndrome as a factor of diminished responsibility or in mitigation then the three criteria for the diagnosis of premenstrual syndrome must be complied with, thus proof is required of:

1. recurrence in each cycle or multiples of each cycle;
2. present in the premenstruum;
3. absence of symptoms in the postmenstruum.

❑ Evidence of menstruation

When a woman is temporarily detained in a police cell there may be evidence that she asked for sanitary protection (see Table 6.3). On the medical examination on admission to prison, records will show the presence or absence of menstruation.

> A 60 year old housewife from St Albans wished to plead that her shoplifting was due to a severe premenstrual migraine attack. On questioning she admitted that it was probably five to seven years since her last menstruation. Naturally, her plea failed and she found another explanation for her behaviour.

> A consultant psychiatrist asked the author to see a 32 year Spanish secretary, who had been diagnosed and successfully treated for premenstrual syndrome some ten years earlier. She had been detained in a South London hospital some six weeks earlier having been found wandering in a confused and rambling state. At

consultation she was alert and produced her diary to confirm that her admission had occurred in the premenstruum. During her alert postmenstruum she had been able to describe her previous illness and treatment, but the psychiatrist found her story unreliable and kept her under observation. Unfortunately a few days before my consultation she had again become confused and rambling, but when menstruation occurred the previous day she had returned to normality once more. At the completion of the interview I reported to the psychiatrist, who was doing a round and was surrounded by the medical registrar and housemen as well as the nursing sister and her juniors, so my report was heard by some twelve individuals. I explained the recent confusion by her being in the premenstruum, but menstruation had started the previous day. The nursing staff disagreed, they insisted her menstruation had occurred twelve days earlier and the recent confusion had occurred in her postmenstruum. The solution appeared simple, inspection of sanitary protection, a vaginal examination or taking a vaginal swab. There were no volunteers to examine the patient, and I was asked to do it. The vaginal swab stained with bright red blood confirmed menstruation and my patient was restarted on appropriate treatment.

This emphasises the importance of proper verification when checking the evidence.

❑ Evidence of recurrence

The diagnosis of premenstrual syndrome requires evidence of recurrence in at least the three preceding menstrual cycles. The mere evidence of recurrent offences in the premenstruum is insufficient in the absence of further corroborative evidence, nevertheless it must be regarded as an indication that further diligent investigation is needed.

A 22 year old woman driver made a plea, at Burnham Bucks, that premenstrual syndrome was the cause of her dangerous driving. She had two crashes in her car each of which was within 48 hours of menstruation on two successive months. Her plea succeeded because there was no one on the prosecution side, or indeed anyone else who was involved in her case, who appreciated the importance of seeking additional evidence, such as any lapses of concentration or instances of aggression in the premenstruums or previous menstrual cycles, or any evidence of superior alertness in the postmenstruum.

The occurrence of two car crashes in the premenstruum could have been a coincidence, and as she pleaded premenstrual syndrome it would have been wise for a treatment order to have been made to remove any danger of further accidents.

On the other hand the mere fact of three shoplifting offences occurring in the premenstruum does not exclude the possibility that the individual is a habitual shoplifter. She may only have been apprehended during her dull, lethargic premenstrual days when she failed to take the necessary precautions to ensure that she was not being observed before removing items from the shelves and placing them in her bag. In her case if she becomes alert in the premenstruum as a result of treatment it may merely make her a better shoplifter, who is not so easily detected.

These two cases illustrate how essential it is that all who are concerned with such pleas, whether in the legal or medical professions, or in any of the ancillary groups involved, are personally fully conversant with the strict criteria of definition, diagnosis and treatment of premenstrual syndrome. It is when there is a lack of such knowledge that the malingerer can abuse the plea. Some women, genuinely handicapped by premenstrual syndrome, will describe the difficulty of returning items inadvertently taken from shops.

It is not necessary for the offence to have been identically the same, nor indeed for an offence to have been committed every month, but the underlying precipitating premenstrual symptoms need to be the same.

P. M. 20 years and unemployed, was charged with assault in a cafe. In evidence she stated that sometimes when alone in her room happily listening to her stereo, she would suddenly get up and smash the set, which was emitting evil sounds. This had occurred on at least six occasions and she was able to produce two receipts giving the dates on which the sets were taken to be repaired.

There was an interval of 30 days between the repair bills, and an interval of 32 days between the date of the last repair bill and the offence with which she had been charged. Thus she was able to successfully prove that cyclical violence had occurred on three consecutive months.

The characteristic of premenstrual syndrome sufferers to have recurrence of offences or similar incidents is discussed on pages 35-36.

❑ Presence in the premenstruum

If there is likely to be any delay before the court appearance it is worth while commencing to keep a menstrual chart immediately. When the woman is confused, amnesic or deluded she will not be able to undertake this task, which should be allocated to a responsible and understanding person.

M. R., a 34 year old housewife, faced two charges of shoplifting, she menstruated on the day of her second charge. She had no idea of her previous dates of the onset of menstruation, but during the four months wait before her trial she produced evidence of cycles of 30-32 days. As the interval between the two alleged offences was 64 days, it was accepted that probably the first offence was also related to menstruation (Figure 11.1).

Trying to accumulate evidence retrospectively is not easy, but it can be done successfully, provided that whatever documents are used have been carefully, accurately and correctly compiled. Particular attention should be given to the precision of timing, which is as important as the event itself and requires as much consideration.

Chris, a 32 year old insurance clerk, lost her temper with her manager from the head office and feared for the loss of her job. She always lost her temper on the last Friday of each month, and was able to bring the exact date of each tantrum, which on the last occasion was exactly two days before the start of menstruation. However, it was only on further questioning that it transpired that the manager only visited her branch office on the last Friday of each month.

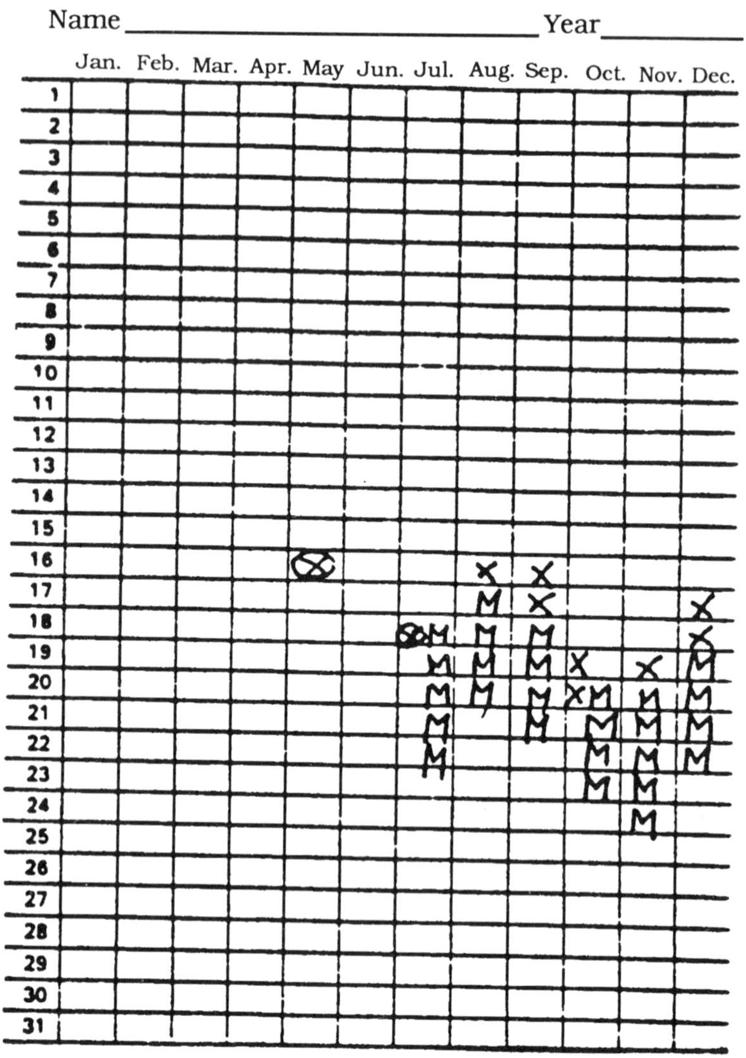

M = menstruation

X = confusion

⊗ = offence

Figure 11.1 Retrospective chart suggesting that both offences occurred in the premenstruum.

Many women keep personal diaries which may contain invaluable information. This information will be more clearly seen when transferred onto a simple menstrual chart together with the dates of menstruation.

The husband of a 47 year old housewife gave evidence that each month there would be a day when he would return home to find his wife had obtained some inappropriate item from the shops, such as dog food, when they had no animals, or baby clothes when their children were almost adults. His wife could never recollect how she obtained the items. He made great efforts to ensure that the car, cash and credit cards were not available during the days at risk. In evidence he showed his diary of the days when he knew precautions would be required. Her plea was successful and progesterone treatment was instituted.

❑ Absence in the postmenstruum

Corroborative evidence can often be found in the increased alertness and intellectual ability of the woman with a surge of activity in the postmenstruum (Dalton 1960 and 1984).

A part time community nurse worked 10 days per month, and chose her duty days with care to avoid the premenstruum knowing full well how confused she would become for a day or two. When a colleague was ill she was called on to work during her premenstruum. In the confusion of her premenstruum she stole a prescription form and forged a prescription for an appetite suppressant. The administrative nursing officer gave evidence on her behalf of the meticulous way she calculated her confused days, which were then taken into account when drawing up each month's rota, but in the emergency produced by her colleague's illness the danger was overlooked. The case was dismissed and progesterone therapy instituted to eliminate the confusion.

❑ Sources of evidence

Careful inspection of other documentation may be helpful in the precise dating of previous incidents of unusual or anti-social behaviour. Police records may reveal dates when a teen-ager went missing or made hoax telephone emergency calls; absences from school or work are usually accurately recorded in the attendance books; medical files and hospital notes may record dates of suicides attempts, wrist slashing or self-mutilation episodes; and prison files record any disorderly conduct. Poison pen writers can usually be timed exactly from the postmark.

The 28 year old barmaid charged with fatally stabbing another barmaid (Chapter 1) was first visited in custody in her prison cell. At the time she could not recall the date of her last menstruation, although she stated that menstruation was regular. Regardless of prompting she was unable to recall how menstruation usually started, as to whether it was scanty or heavy on the first day, whether it was painful or accompanied by backache or if the initial loss was pink, red, brown or black. Such genuine blankness about the onset of menstruation may be a sign of temporary amnesia and confusion. However, her prison records showed she was menstruating on admission to prison a few hours after the fatal stabbing. Inspection of her prison records revealed that although she was described by medical officers as 'pleasant and cooperative, apart from episodes of attention-seeking behaviour', even these episodes were occurring at regular intervals (Figure 11.2) (Dalton 1980).

She had 26 previous convictions for which she had served prison sentences. A further search of her prison documents revealed that there were 25 episodes of violence in prison, which had been reported to the prison governor. With a statisticians's assistance the dates of these episodes of violence were analysed and found to have occurred in cycles of 29.55 ± 1.45 days (Dalton 1980) (Figure 11.3).

Furthermore, the days of committing her offences, for which she had previously been sentenced, showed the

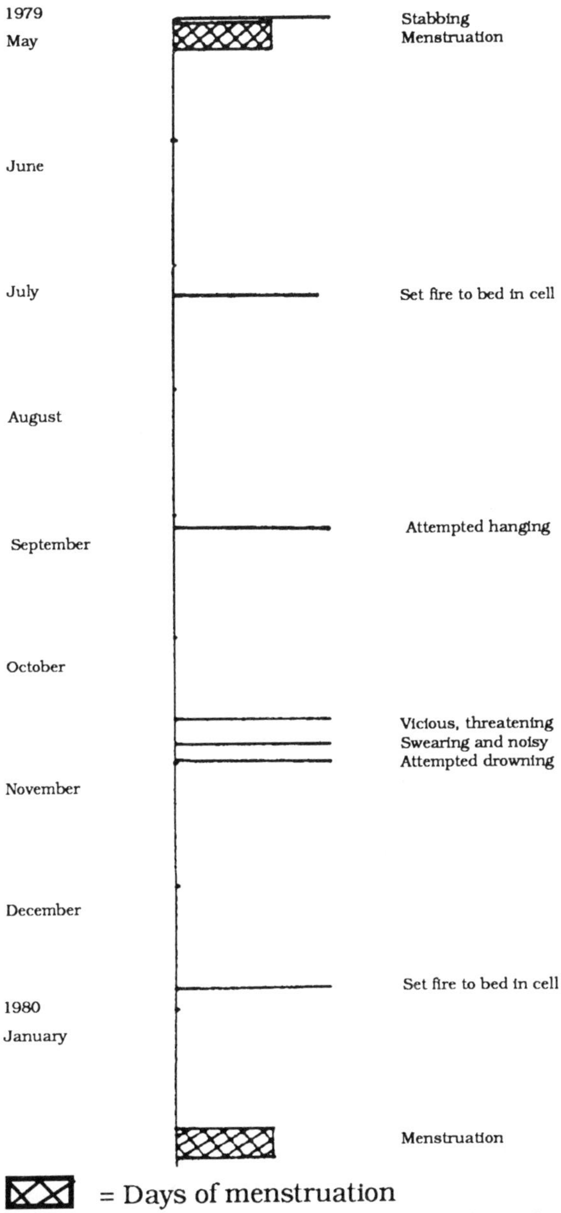

Figure 11.2 Timing of offences while in prison relative to menstruation. *From 'Behaviour and the Menstrual Cycle', Ed. Friedman R. C. (1983) Dalton K. Chapter 11.*

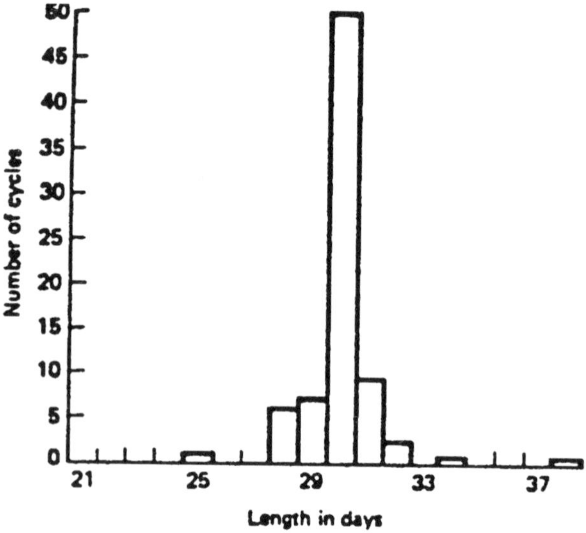

Figure 11.3 Distribution of 'fitted' cycles between episodes of violence in prison. *From Dalton K. (1980) Lancet.*

> average cycle length, which could be fitted in between the offences was 29.04 ± 1.47 days (Figure 11.4).
>
> It was on the basis of these findings that a diagnosis of premenstrual syndrome was made. The judge allowed sentence to be postponed for five months during which her response to progesterone therapy was observed. As there were no further episodes of bad behaviour, she was released on probation with an order to continue treatment.

Another example where successful retrospective search required scrutiny from many sources of information was that of an 18 year old student (Dalton 1980).

> The student had been of exemplary behaviour, winning many prizes, until menstruation started at 13 years, but during the following year she had episodes of strange behaviour which her parents could not understand. On one occasion she set fire to the bedroom curtains. After an interval she ran away from home and was returned by

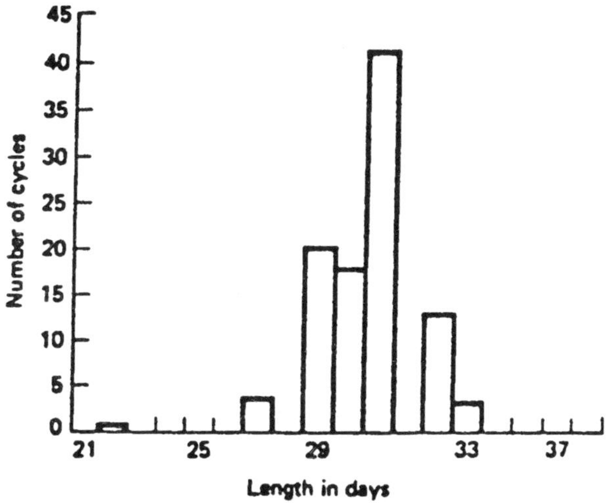

Figure 11.4 Distribution of 'fitted' cycles between prison admissions. *From Dalton K. (1980) Lancet 1081.*

the police. Later she unexpectedly shaved her head and eyebrows as she felt so ugly; a few weeks later she slashed her fingers and sought help from the local hospital. The precise dates of these episodes were obtained by finding the date of the insurance claim for the burnt curtains; information from the local police; the date of the cheque when the parents bought her a wig to cover her shaven head; and the date the casualty officer sutured her fingers. These events occurred at intervals of 28-32 days, although the dates of menstruation were unknown. Two years later she committed arson and was immediately taken into custody where records showed she was menstruating on admission to prison. Within days she was released on bail, but a month later she was charged with being drunk and disorderly while on bail. She was returned to prison and again it was noted that she was menstruating. She was again released on bail, but a month later she took an overdose and had a short hospital stay, the hospital notes stated she was menstruating. After three months there was another more serious fire at her father's house, she was again committed to prison and was noted to be menstruating. The following month, while still in prison, she slashed her wrists and the next day tried to strangle herself by fixing a sheet to the top of the window. She was again menstruating. This retrospective information was used to confirm the diagnosis of premenstrual syndrome. She received progesterone treatment, experienced normal menstruation and was released on probation (Dalton 1980). Now ten years later she is leading a normal, happy life with a successful career, although still receiving progesterone therapy.

In the appeal of *R v Reynolds* against a life sentence for the murder of her mother it was scrutiny of the judge's summing up, which produced the evidence of premenstrual syndrome.

A student of 18 years lived alone with her mother. She became pregnant, and to keep her pregnancy secret she moved to another town, gave birth to a boy on 11th April 1986 and had him adopted immediately. She returned home within a few days and returned to college, taking her 'A' level examinations as normal, and at the end of term took two part time jobs. On 28th June she murdered her mother with a hammer, and was immediately taken to the police station. She was there examined by Dr. H de la H Davies, the police surgeon, who made the diagnosis of depression and premenstrual tension.

In his summing up the Honourable Mr. Justice Tudor-Evans reminded the jury that Dr. Kinnerley, her general practitioner, was called to the house on 11th May as the defendant was menstruating heavily. She had told her mother about her pregnancy and stated 'I felt I was going to pieces... I thought I would just walk out... I felt I was cracking'. One does not know when the vaginal bleeding started, but it is worth noting that she was menstruating 30 days after baby's birth. The judge also reminded the jury that on June 1st the defendant had planned to stay with her boy friend's mother, but telephoned and 'said she was not well'. Note this is precisely 27 days before the killing.

The judge reminded the jury that Dr. O'Connor, psychiatrist, did not 'think there was clinical depression on July 3rd, that came about three weeks later'. Thus she was not depressed in the postmenstruum when Dr. O'Connor first saw her on July 3rd, but she became depressed three weeks later during the subsequent premenstruum or menstruation. The diagnosis of premenstrual syndrome was further confirmed by her low SHBG estimation. She was released on probation with a two year treatment order (Table 11.1).

Table 11.1 Evidence from the Judge's summing up *R. v Reynolds*

1986	
April 11	Baby born.
May 11	Heavy menstruation, doctor called.
June 1	Unwell, unable to go away.
June 28	Mother killed, defendant menstruating.
July 3	First consultation with psychiatrist, defendant not depressed.
July 24*	Psychiatrist diagnosed depression, not present 3 weeks earlier.

* = estimated date

❑ Testing the evidence

The statements made by defendants should not all be taken at face value. Shoplifters should be asked in confidence of other items they might have taken accidentally, what their reaction had been, and whether or not they had tried to return the items. Sometimes it is even possible to put the evidence to the test.

F. W. 30 year old air hostess, was charged with driving under the influence of alcohol, having a blood alcohol level of 140 mg/l. She attributed this raised level to being in her premenstruum and being the last day of the course of an oestrogen-progestogen oral contraceptive. Her story was that she had a gin and tonic at 18.00 hours at home, then a steak and salad supper and a further gin and tonic at 19.00 hours. She was only an occasional social drinker, but took a drink that night knowing it would help her sleep as she was due to report for work at 3.00 hours the next morning. However, she received a phone call from her ex-fiance and decided to drive instead to London, a journey of $1^1/_2$ hours. Arriving at his flat she found no one at home so drove back. At 23.30 hours she was noticed to be driving erratically, and was stopped by police and breathalysed. The incident occurred on the last day of her course of the pill and two days before menstruation started. She could not understand how she could possibly have had such a high blood alcohol level, only having had two gin and tonics $5^1/_2$ hours earlier. It seemed easy enough to test this story, and it was planned to test the blood alcohol level in her premenstruum and postmenstruum, both on and off the pill. The first test was on the last day of her course of the pill and two days before menstruation, when the blood level would be expected to be at its highest. Supervised throughout by the doctor's secretary, she had an initial blood alcohol test, took a gin and tonic, had a steak and salad meal, a further glass of gin and tonic and five and a half hours later had a second blood alcohol test. The second blood test showed a blood alcohol well below the maximum level so plans for further tests were abandoned. She must have drunk more alcohol on the day of the incident than she could recall. She lost her licence for one year and was fined £100.

❑ Diagnostic pointers

The presence of positive diagnostic pointers are valuable additional evidence for the diagnosis of premenstrual syndrome, but there must still be evidence that the event occurred in the premenstruum. The Diagnostic Check List Score is discussed on pages 53-57.

In Britain the most valuable source of factual information are the medical records, which are transferred from one general practitioner to the other when the patient moves around the country. In addition to recording any previous consultations and medication for premenstrual syndrome the records may also note side effects on the pill; adult weight swings; the presence of threatened abortion, preeclampsia or postnatal depression; suicide attempts or self mutilation; previous psychiatric consultations or sterilisation. However, factual evidence is still required so it is still necessary to obtain a hospital report of a suicide attempt, or a consultant's evidence of postnatal depression or sterilisation. In such cases the patient must give written permission for the information to be disclosed.

❑ Reference

Dalton K. (1980). *Lancet*, **2**, 1070-1071.
Dalton K. (1982). *'Behavior and the Menstrual Cycle'*. Ed: Friedman R.C., Marcel Dekker Inc.: New York. Chapter 11, 217-242.

12

Aetiology of Premenstrual Syndrome

"Aetiology is an inquiry in to the origin or causes of anything, especially a disease". (Chambers Twentieth Century Dictionary). Before discussing the aetiology it is useful to bring together the known facts about premenstrual syndrome, because any aetiological theory must embrace these facts. Premenstrual syndrome is:

1. A disease that affects women – only during their child-bearing years.
2. It is present in the premenstruum when progesterone is required during the luteal phase.
3. It is absent in the postmenstruum when progesterone is not required during the follicular phase.
4. It is absent in pregnancy when the blood level of progesterone is very high (Figure 4.3).
5. It is worse after pregnancy, when the body is suddenly deprived of the high and continuous level of progesterone.

Other factors to be taken into consideration are:

6. Cyclical premenstrual syndrome symptoms can continue after removal of the uterus and/or both ovaries, therefore the cause of premenstrual syndrome does not lie in the uterus or ovaries alone.
7. Premenstrual syndrome characteristically starts at a time of marked alterations of progesterone levels, such as occurs at puberty, with the pill, after a pregnancy, cessation of menstruation and after sterilisation (pages 48-49).
8. Increase in severity of symptoms of premenstrual syndrome occurs after a hormonal event in which there was a marked alteration of progesterone level (pages 48-49).
9. Women with premenstrual syndrome are unable to tolerate long intervals without food and/or have food binges (pages 52-53).

10. Women with premenstrual syndrome are unable to tolerate the pill or the artificial progestogens, which lower the blood progesterone level (pages 50-51).
11. Complete relief of premenstrual syndrome occurs with the correct dose of progesterone.

These facts suggest that premenstrual syndrome is a hormone disorder as opposed to a disease of the mind, and more specifically these facts suggest that premenstrual syndrome is a disease involving progesterone.

❑ Progesterone hormonal pathway

> "No phenomenon or stage in a sequence has only one cause: all antecedent stages are successive causes and as science has no reason to infer a first cause, the sequence of causes can be carried back to the limit of knowledge."

These words, from *'The Grammar of Science'* (1892) by Walter Scott quoted in the *British Medical Journal* (Macfarlane 1984), would also apply to the aetiology of premenstrual syndrome and its relationship to progesterone.

The varying levels of progesterone in the blood during the menstrual cycle and in pregnancy has already been discussed (Chapter 4 and Figure 4.2).

Progesterone has a complicated hormonal pathway (Figure 12.1). Much consideration will be needed to determine exactly where the fault may lie. It is not necessarily the same site for all sufferers; indeed it is more probable that the actual site of the progesterone inadequacy differs in different women.

The effect of stress in altering the times of menstruation has already been discussed (pages 26-28) (Dalton 1968). Stress would act by increasing stimuli being received by the *cerebrum*.

The fault could lie in the *hypothalamus* at the base of the brain where the menstrual controlling centre is situated. This is now known to be a collection of areas which interact one with another to control *gonadotrophin* release, along with many other functions such as the control of weight and day/night rhythm. The hypothalamus is situated near the floor of the third ventricle which is filled with cerebro-spinal fluid. There

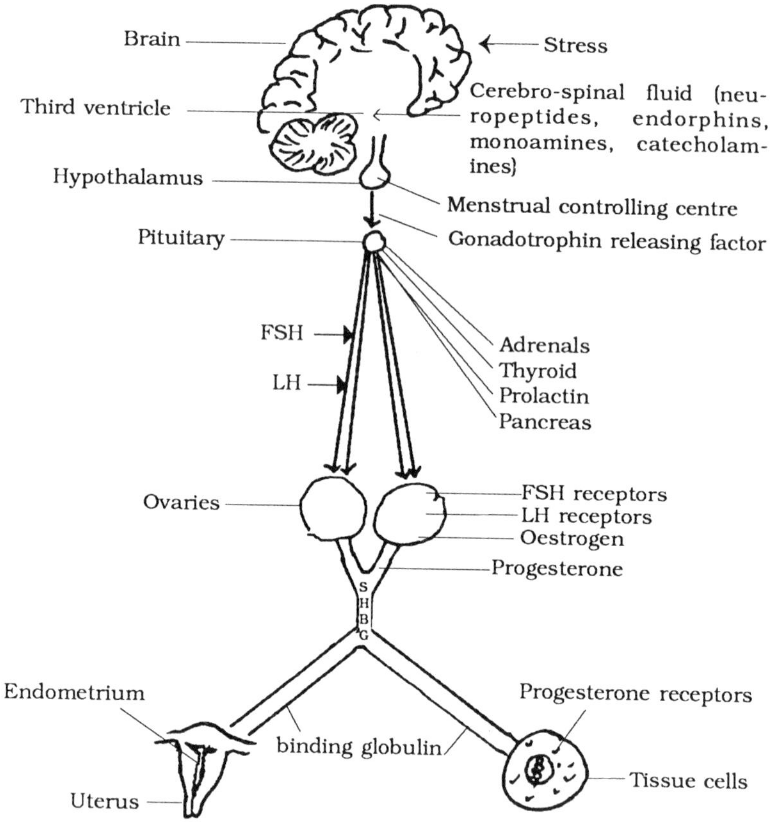

Figure 12.1 Progesterone hormonal pathway

are special cells, known as *tanycytes*, which have ciliated cell bodies lining the floor of the third ventricle and ending in the portal system of the hypothalamus (Spiroff *et al* 1983). These cells pass information about the composition of the cerebrospinal fluid to the hypothalamus. Thus substances found in the cerebrospinal fluid, such as neuropeptides, endorphins, monoamines, catecholamines, serotonin, and pineal fluid secretion will all affect gonadotrophin release. It has recently been suggested that endorphins or alphamelanocyte stimulating hormone (α MSH) secretion may moderate the mood and behaviour changes of premenstrual syndrome (Reid and Yen 1981).

The *pituitary* has been described as 'the leader of the body's hormonal orchestra', for in addition to synthesising numerous different hormones it also receives input from the hormones of the ovaries, adrenals, thyroid, pancreas, and renin-angeotension-aldosterone axis which in turn affect the levels of FSH and LH, either increasing or decreasing the levels.

❑ The ovary

The stimulus of FSH from the pituitary acting on the ovarian tissue causes the maturation of an immature ovum, or egg cell, and also stimulates the production of oestrogen, which acts on the uterus. The stimulus of LH from the pituitary acting on the ovary causes ovulation, release of the ovum, and leads to the production of progesterone.

❑ Progesterone

Progesterone is the oldest steroid known and is present in all vertebrates, such as birds, snakes, rodents, dogs, horses, and apes. Not all vertebrates menstruate and in the lower vertebrates the function of progesterone is limited to sugar metabolism and intelligence (Elias 1986), as well as being a building block in the formation of cortical steroids. It is only in the higher vertebrates that progesterone is involved in reproduction and menstruation. For obvious reasons brain biopsies are not available from healthy individuals to compare with premenstrual syndrome sufferers, so for the moment one must rely on the findings from animal studies. It is the molecular biologists, who have studied the characteristics of progesterone and progesterone receptors in lower vertebrates, and revealed invaluable clues as to the behaviour of progesterone receptors *in vitro*.

❑ Hormone binding

Progesterone needs to be transported in the blood to the cells where it is to be utilised. Both progesterone and oestrogen are transported by being bound in the plasma to specific binding proteins and non-specific binding proteins such as albumin

(Spiroff *et al* 1983). Progesterone is bound to cortisol binding globulin (CBG, previously called transcortin) which also binds cortisol. Careful control is needed to maintain free cortisol levels within the desired range of the body. Therefore, one would not expect to find major alterations in the cortisol binding globulin levels in patients with premenstrual syndrome, because they would also then show changes in cortisol metabolism. Oestradiol is bound to sex hormone binding globulin (SHBG) which also binds testosterone and has an even higher affinity to dihydrotestosterone. Changes in SHBG levels alter oestradiol and testosterone levels and, as testosterone binds to SHBG with a greater affinity, changes in SHBG levels reflect greater changes in oestradiol levels. SHBG binding capacity is low in premenstrual syndrome (Dalton M. E. 1981). Progesterone raises the binding capacity of SHBG, whereas the artificial progestogens lower the binding capacity (Dalton M. E. 1984). (See pages 59-62).

❑ Hormone receptors

Hormone receptors are situated within cells and their task is to transfer a molecule of the hormone from the cell substance, over the nuclear wall and into the nucleus attaching the hormone molecule to the DNA, where it can be metabolised and utilised. Hormone receptors are very specific and only act for one hormone. There appear to be hormones receptors for all the common hormones, such as thyroid, cortisone, oestrogen, FSH and LH, but our concern is with the progesterone receptors.

❑ Sites of progesterone receptors

The progesterone in the blood can only be utilised by cells which contain progesterone receptors. Studies suggest that the largest accumulation of progesterone receptors is in the mid-brain, the limbic area, which is the area referred to by animal biologists as the 'centre of rage and violence' (Figure 12.2).

A study of the distribution of progesterone receptors (Figure 12.2) shows the relationship of the sites of progesterone

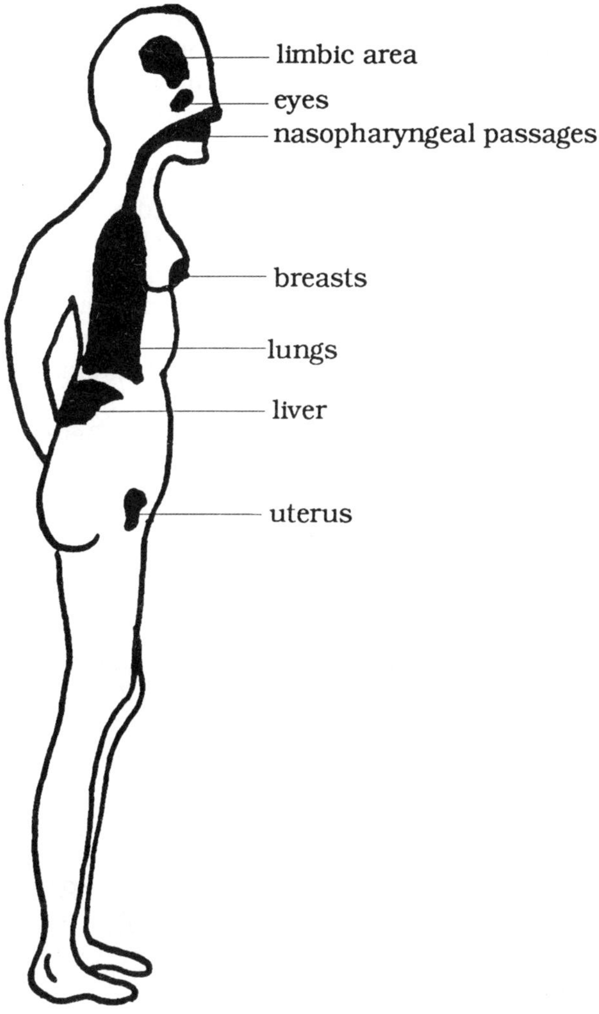

Figure 12.2 Sites of progesterone receptors

receptors to the other premenstrual syndrome symptoms, which are the eyes, nasopharyngeal passages, lungs, breasts, liver and uterus. There are also many progesterone receptors in the hypothalamus and preoptic area which account for the distribution of premenstrual headaches, which tend to be centred in the forehead and around the eyes where many progesterone receptors are found (Figure 12.3) (Dalton 1984). This is in contrast to the distribution of tension headaches, which occur in men and women and are caused by tension and stress, for in tension headaches the pain is essentially occipital or vertical and the pain radiates down the neck.

If progesterone is administered orally it passes via the portal system to the liver where it is inactivated by the progesterone receptors before it has a chance to reach the systemic circulation and limbic areas, eyes, nasopharyngeal passages, lungs, breasts and uterus. This is the explanation why natural progesterone needs to be administered intramuscularly, vaginally or rectally but not orally. On the other hand, the artificial progestogens, such as are contained in the oral contraceptives, are alien to the human body and therefore have no specific receptors. They cannot be utilised by the progesterone receptors in the liver and so pass into the systemic circulation to reach the uterus.

❑ Characteristics of progesterone receptors

Two characteristics of the behaviour of progesterone receptors are relevant to the understanding of progesterone treatment

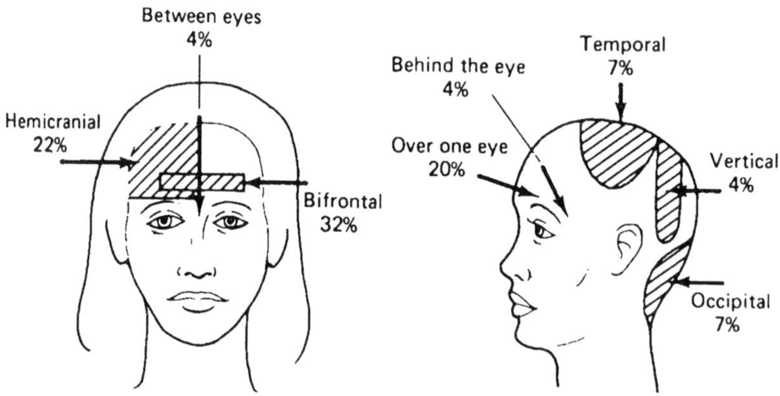

Figure 12.3 Sites of pain in premenstrual headaches. *From Dalton K. (1984) 'Premenstrual Syndrome and Progesterone Therapy', 2nd Edition.*

for premenstrual syndrome, and only these characteristics will be described.

When the first dose of progesterone is administered to a rat's hypothalamus there is a rapid movement of progesterone receptors from the cytoplasm, or cell substance, into the nuclei of the cells (Blaustein 1987). However when the next dose is administered there is no such movement until the dose of progesterone is increased forty fold. Thus the progesterone receptors are not insensitive to a second or higher dose, but they are hyposensitive. Naturally one wonders the reason for the hyposensitivity, and one suggestion is related to the progesterone blood level in pregnancy when the placenta produces vast amounts of progesterone, so much that the blood level of progesterone may reach more than forty times the level present at the peak in the menstrual cycle (pages 22-23). This high level of placental progesterone is essentially for the benefit of the developing fetus and it may be that there is a built-in blocking mechanism to ensure priority of progesterone for the fetus and only excess progesterone is made available for the mother. This would explain why premenstrual syndrome is so much worse after a pregnancy or after cessation of menstruation, as the blockade by progesterone receptors may continue when menstruation is resumed. It also explains why such large doses of progesterone are needed in treatment.

❑ Blood sugar levels

Before discussing the other characteristic of progesterone receptors it is necessary to understand the body's control of blood sugar levels, for the blood sugar level has to be maintained between strict optimum levels and to ensure this there is an upper and lower self-regulating mechanism. If excess sugar enters the blood and the blood sugar level rises too high the upper regulating mechanism acts by increasing insulin and passing the excess sugar into the urine, thus restoring the blood sugar level within the optimum range. On the other hand, if the blood sugar level is too low it is the lower regulating mechanism that comes into action with a spurt of adrenalin, which serves to release the sugar stored in the body's cells, which then passes into the blood. Thus the blood sugar level is constantly maintained within optimum range. Normally a woman can go 4 to 6 hours before her blood sugar level drops so low that it triggers a spurt of adrenalin (Figure 12.4). Men can go longer, about 7 to 8 hours. The level of the lower regulating mechanism is raised during the premenstruum, especially in sufferers of premenstrual syndrome, the effect of this is that her blood sugar level will trigger the lower regulating mechanism bringing it into action after a shorter interval of about 3 hours without carbohydrate intake, so causing spurts of adrenalin to occur more frequently (Figure 12.4).

The sugar in the blood comes from the breakdown of the carbohydrates that are eaten. There are two types of carbohydrates. The simple ones are the sugars (glucose, fructose and sucrose), which when eaten cause a rapid rise, followed by an equally rapid drop in blood sugar level. The complex carbohydrates are the starches, like flour, potatoes, rice, oats or rye, which when eaten cause a more gradual rise in blood sugar level and then a more gradual drop in blood sugar level. In a normal woman if there is a gap of five or six hours in the

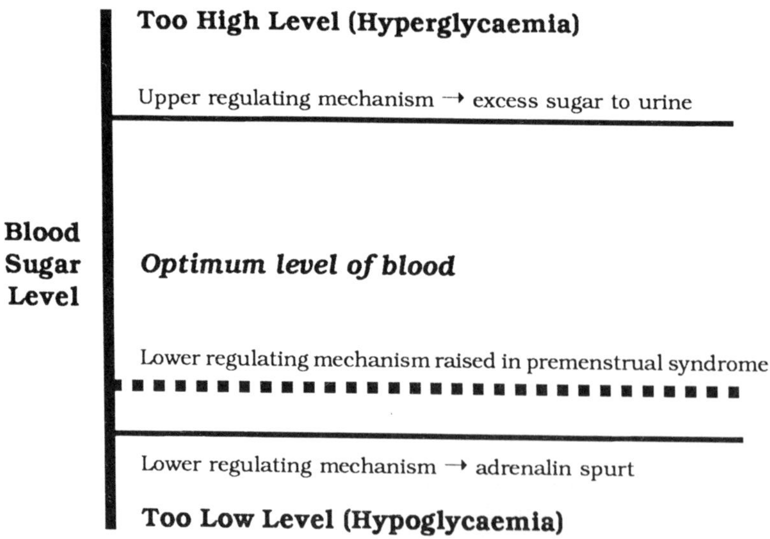

Figure 12.4 Control mechanism for blood sugar.

daytime when no starch containing food is eaten the level of her blood sugar falls and the lower regulating mechanism is activated, causing spurts of adrenalin until more sugar or starch is eaten (Figure 12.5).

Adrenalin is the hormone of fight, flight, and fright, and it is this accumulation of adrenalin which is responsible for the sudden explosive outbursts, the out-of-control irritability, panics, and confusion which may occur in premenstrual syndrome.

❑ Progesterone receptors and adrenalin

Returning to the other characteristics of progesterone receptors, it has been shown in rodents that progesterone receptors do not transport molecules of progesterone into the nuclei of cells in the presence of adrenalin (Nock 1987), and adrenalin

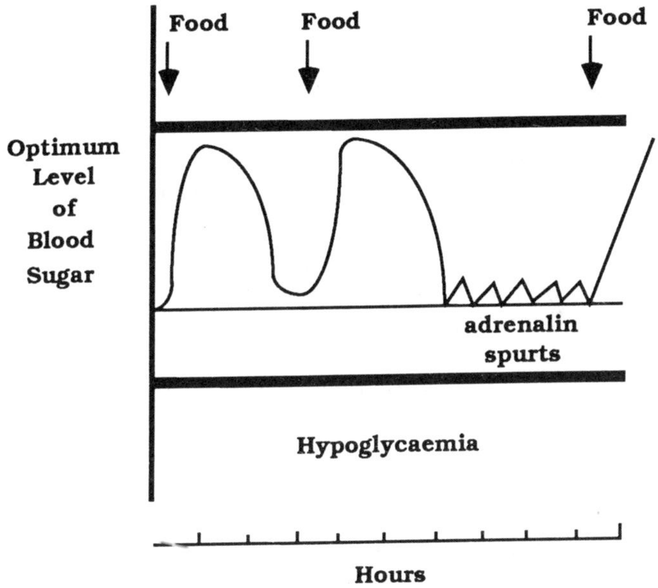

Figure 12.5 Effect of long food interval during the premenstruum in a premenstrual syndrome patient.

is released when the blood sugar level drops. Thus when premenstrual syndrome sufferers go too long without carbohydrates the adrenalin prevents the uptake of progesterone by the progesterone receptors. It will have been noted how often in the reported case histories (pages 56-57) mention is made of the long interval the sufferer went without food preceding the episode of confusion, amnesia or violence, which resulted in her court appearance. The importance of this finding lies in the necessity in treatment not only to correct the sufferer's progesterone balance, but also to ensure that she is having sufficient carbohydrate during waking hours to prevent the release of adrenalin.

Adrenalin is also produced at times of stress and this suggests why premenstrual syndrome is worse at times of stress.

There are many areas where a fault in the progesterone pathway may occur in premenstrual syndrome, and research is constantly being undertaken to unravel the mysteries of premenstrual syndrome in different women. However, there is no excuse to hold up the precise diagnosis or effective treatment which eliminates distressing symptoms.

❑ References

Blaustein J.D. (1986). *Reproduction: A Behavioural and Neusoendocrine Prospective;* Ed. Komusaruk B. R. Annals New York Acad Sci, New York.

Dalton K. (1968). *Lancet 2,* 1386-1388.

Dalton K. (1984). *The Premenstrual Syndrome and Progesterone Therapy* William Heinemann Med Bks, London/Year Book Med Pub. Chicago.

Dalton M.E. (1981). *Postgrad Med J;* **57**, 560-561

Dalton M.E. (1984). *J. Ster, Biochem;* Jan.

Elia I. (1985). *The Female Animal;* Oxford University Press, Oxford.

Macfarlane A. (1984). *Brit Med J.;* **289**, 6457, 1473.

Nock (1986). *Reproduction: A Behavioural and Neurological Prospective;* Ed Komusaruk B. R. Annals New York Acad Sci. New York.

Reid R.L. & Yen S.S.C. (1981). *Amer. J. Obstet Gynec;* 139, 1, 85-104.
Spiroff L. Glass R.H. & Kose N.G. (1983) *Clinical Endocrinology and Infertility;* Williams and Wilkins, Baltimore/London.

13

Treatment of Premenstrual Syndrome

The effect of severe premenstrual syndrome is often wretched, frequently distressing and occasionally tragic, but it does have the redeeming feature that once it has been correctly diagnosed and proper treatment instituted a return to normal health is assured as long as treatment is monitored and maintained.

Treatment is essential for any women whose premenstrual syndrome is so severe that they are brought before the court. One has only to consider the American mother of six children arrested for battering one of her children and who claimed premenstrual syndrome in her defence. She had no treatment, yet asked the judge to release her presumably so that she could batter her children in the following premenstruums. In England evidence of successful treatment, or agreement to submit to treatment is frequent, and should be included in the probation order, for society must be protected from the possible harm which can be caused by sufferers of untreated severe premenstrual syndrome.

Unquestionably a correct diagnosis is the first step in the treatment of any and every disease, but how do we decide what is the right treatment for that disease? Surely it must be those treatments which are able to restore normality in the patient and maintain normality over the years with a minimum of side effects. Today, the correct treatment for premenstrual syndrome is being obscured by too many commercial interests marketing a plethora of nutritional products, vitamins and minerals. This chapter deals with a treatment schedule that has been successfully used to bring normality to thousands of premenstrual syndrome sufferers for over forty years, and has no long term or short term side effects and is the treatment ordered by the courts in serious premenstrual syndrome based offences. The treatment is with the natural hormone, progesterone. The previous chapter provides an understanding for this treatment.

Many estimates have been made as to the number of women suffering from premenstrual syndrome. The figures vary according to the definition used and range from 30% to 90%, but these are guesswork for none of the studies on which the estimates were based have used the strict criteria for the definition of premenstrual syndrome, which was set out in Chapter 5. Using this definition, it can fairly reasonably be estimated that about 40% of all menstruating women suffer from premenstrual syndrome at some time in their menstruating years. Some 10- 20% will have it mildly, in perhaps another 10-20% it will be of moderate severity and a further 10% will suffer severely. This 10% of severe sufferers can be broken down further to reveal the offenders, who probably represent little more than 1% of severe sufferers. It is estimated that 90% of that group are as yet unrecognised, which leaves, at present, only a minute group that are known and treated. It should be noted that there are shaded areas in Figure 13.1, this is to emphasise that the proportions are only approximate, for there are no clear boundaries, no firm details of the numbers of sufferers.

Those whose premenstrual syndrome is of such severity as to bring them into court and those with symptoms suggestive of criminal potential deserve and need treatment. The treatment is three pronged and includes (1) hormone therapy, (2) dietary advice and (3) education.

❑ The Drug of Choice

In cases of severe premenstrual syndrome the question of definitive hormone therapy arises. The drug must be able to raise the blood progesterone level and also the SHBG level (Dalton 1984), this occurs with natural progesterone, whereas the artificial progestogens (see pages 50-51) lower both the blood progesterone level and also the SHBG level.

The drug must not stop menstruation, as studies have shown that when menstruation is stopped there is an increase in the severity of premenstrual syndrome with the restarting of menstruation. Therefore oestrogen implants, which stop menstruation, are contraindicated. Oestrogen stimulates the

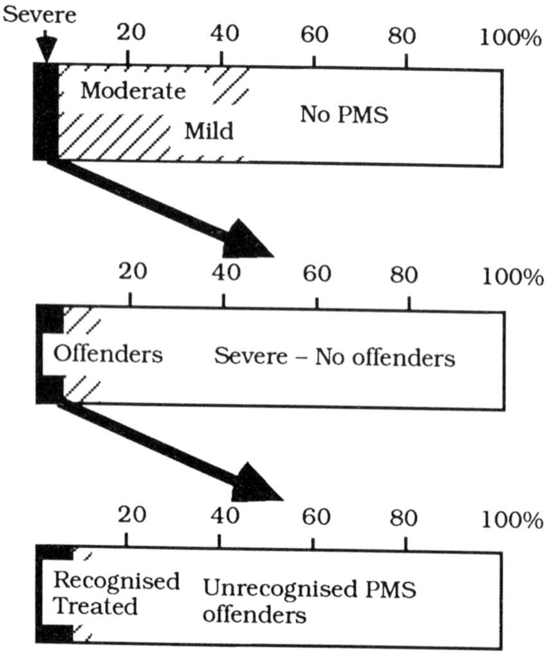

Figure 13.1 Estimated incidence of premenstrual syndrome offenders.

lining of the womb, so when using oestrogen it is essential to have regular shedding of the lining to prevent a build-up of tissue which might be dangerous. This regular bleeding is usually achieved by giving a progestogen for a few days each month. Magos and his colleagues (1986) have noted that when women, who had received an oestrogen implant, were given progestogens cyclically they developed typical premenstrual syndrome symptoms each month.

Drugs with known side effects should be avoided, as women do not wish to lose some symptoms only to develop different distressing symptoms. So drugs such as Danol and the new LHRH agonists which may cause weight gain, masculinsation, nausea, vertigo or amenorrhoea are best avoided. Addictive drugs should not be used for a chronic condition such as premenstrual syndrome, so the benzodiazepams must be rigorously avoided.

In short the best treatment for severe premenstrual syndrome is progesterone, but it needs to be used together with dietary advice and education (Table 13.2).

Table 13.2 Schedule of Treatment for Premenstrual Syndrome

Premenstrual syndrome diagnosed

Progesterone	Diet	Education
Individual tailoring Suppository Pessary Injection	3 hourly starchy food throughout menstrual cycle	stop pill avoid sterilisation stop night work avoid progestogens stop vitamin B6

❑ Progesterone Therapy

As this book is written for non-medical professional readers only the principles of progesterone treatment will be given. The medical profession, which administers and monitors treatment, has its own sources of more detailed information (Dalton 1984).

Progesterone has been consistently used for the treatment of premenstrual syndrome since 1948. It was first reported in the British Medical Journal in 1953 by Greene and Dalton, who reported that 85% of women suffering from premenstrual syndrome were made symptomfree and a further 8% improved on progesterone. The success depends on meticulous diagnosis and individual tailoring (Dalton 1984). If the patient does not have menstrual distress, and the diagnosis of premenstrual syndrome is confirmed then failure to improve is due to incorrect dosage, usually too low a dose or failure to absorb rectally or vaginally, or to not having tried intramuscular injections.

As long ago as 1958 a Tribunal on Overprescribing in General

Practice agreed that 'progesterone is reasonable and necessary treatment for premenstrual syndrome', and ever since general practitioners have been able to prescribe progesterone without fear of being charged with overprescribing.

The Food and Drug Administration of America in February 1983 approved progesterone for the treatment of premenstrual syndrome as far as safety was concerned, but demanded dose ranging clinical trials to prove the efficacy. In Britain, progesterone injections and progesterone suppositories have been licenced by the Committee of Safety of Medicines for many years, which means that production is quality controlled. On the other hand until progesterone suppositories are passed by the American Food and Drug Administration for efficiency there is no quality control, and each individual will have to rely on her own pharmacy. Recently it was found that some progesterone suppositories marketed in America purporting to contain 400mg were found to contain only 238 mg on analysis.

❑ Progesterone is prophylactic

Progesterone therapy needs to be started before any symptoms of premenstrual syndrome have occurred. The usual course is from ovulation until menstruation. Different women have different absorptive capacities for progesterone. Some absorb quickly, but then the level drops quickly. Others absorb slowly, and the level may last longer. About 10% of sufferers do not absorb sufficiently from the rectum or vagina and require intramuscular injections (Dalton 1984).

❑ Principles of Progesterone Therapy

Very high levels of progesterone occur naturally during pregnancy, and the woman's body is designed to cope with these levels (Figure 4.3). With our present methods of progesterone administration, it is impossible to reach progesterone blood levels much higher than would naturally occur at about the 12th to 16th week of pregnancy. This means that there is no risk of an overdose with progesterone administered intramuscularly, rectally or vaginally. Even those who have previously abused drugs, can safely be given extra suppositories to use if they require it. If two suppositories are used in the same orifice at the same time, the accumulated wax will prevent further absorption. It is advisable to wait about two hours between administrations.

Progesterone is a natural hormone, and there are no drug reactions if used with other drugs. However, if the patient is on the pill or taking progestogens, it is best to stop them as all progestogens lower the blood progesterone level. After all, there is no point in giving progesterone to raise the blood progesterone level if, at the same time, the progestogens are lowering it. If women are already on anti-depressants or tranquillisers, these can initially be continued at the normal dose until the progesterone begins to take effect and then the dose of tranquillisers can gradually be reduced each postmenstruum.

There are no contra-indications to progesterone, although in women with a monilial infection (yeast or thrush) suppositories may cause an exacerbation of moniliasis. If moniliasis is present it should first be treated in both the patient and her partner before using progesterone vaginally. If there is a history of colitis or faecal incontinence, progesterone is best administered vaginally. Occasionally progesterone may lengthen or shorten a cycle; this can be corrected by dose adjustment. Rarely, there may be generalised urticarial reaction from the ethyl oleate in which the progesterone injection is dissolved. In such cases, treatment can be continued by suppositories.

❑ Personal tailoring

It is necessary to personally tailor each patient's progesterone therapy. Factors to be taken into consideration include the varying length of cycle, duration of flow and day of heaviest loss, number of pregnancies and any complications, severity, timing and type of symptoms, patients' ability to absorb progesterone and the contraceptive needs. Those who require daily supervision during the premenstruum are started on injections. This enables the community nurse to visit the patient at home daily to give the injection and at the same time silently supervise her condition and report any deterioration.

❑ Lapsed treatment

A course of progesterone at the right dose given from ovulation until menstruation removes premenstrual symptoms for that cycle. Treatment must therefore be repeated month by month to prevent a recurrence of symptoms. Difficulties arise when a woman is released from prison before arrangements are made for her own doctor to be informed of her treatment or before he is able to procure a supply of progesterone. In these cases a recurrence is likely to occur within a few days of release (Dalton 1980). It is valuable for the probation order to be conditional upon a continuation of treatment. In one case not only did the order demand that she continues with her daily progesterone injections, but also laid on the nurse the responsibility to sign daily that the defendant had eaten every three hours during the previous day.

> S. C. missed her daily injections on two occasions. The first due to an administrative error, when the daily nurse was ill and the deputy was not sent for four days. On the second occasion, when she was gradually being reduced from daily injections to suppositories, it later transpired that she did not use the suppositories. On both occasions, there was a further infringement of the law within a matter of days, both of which resulted in an extension of the probation order, which has now expired after three years.

It is also necessary for the general practitioner to appreciate the need for continuation of progesterone treatment, and the need for gradual reduction before final cessation.

> Miss M. W., an unemployed 19 year old from Cornwall, had responded well to progesterone following her imprisonment for causing grievous bodily harm. After six months, when she was very well and free from symptoms, her doctor abruptly stopped treatment, only to find her violent behaviour was again repeated the following month.

Those who move about the country, as is frequently the case in today's mobile society, are apt to stop treatment. A new doctor sees them, assesses their normality in the postmenstruum, and without a full background knowledge decides on some other medication, usually tranquillisers or anti-depressants and before long she is in trouble once again. For these few women it may be wise to give a progesterone implant, which provides a base progesterone level for a few months, even if it interferes with the normal menstrual rhythm. Implantation also provides a continuous supply of progesterone throughout the whole of the menstrual cycle whereas normally it is present only in the luteal phase.

❑ Dietary advice

The findings of the animal biologists, that progesterone receptors are unable to pick up molecules of progesterone in the presence of adrenalin (see Chapter 11), emphasises the importance of a starch diet for sufferers of premenstrual syndrome. The maxim is to eat little and often, ensuring that they have small portions of starchy food every three hours. The starchy foods are those containing:

Flour e. g. bread, biscuits, pizza, pasta, pancakes and custard
Potatoes including roast, baked, boiled, jacket and crisps
Rice, boiled, cakes and biscuits
Oats, porridge, cakes and flapjacks
Rye, bread and crispbreads.

This does not mean eating more food, but it does mean dividing the normal daily food intake into six meals and ensuring that each half-meal contains some starchy food. This can be achieved by halving the amount of toast or cereal at breakfast and having the other half with mid-morning coffee; halving the starchy food at lunch so that the other half can be eaten at mid-afternoon; and saving the starchy dessert from supper to eat before retiring. It is quite simple and if already on a good diet it does not entail eating any extra food, so there's no need to worry about gaining weight. Self discipline is also required to avoid the temptation of eating six full meals each day.

One has to develop the habit of eating little and often throughout the whole menstrual cycle, as well as on holidays and festivities. So one needs to ensure that there is always a small snack handy, such as a packet of biscuits readily available in the handbag or car to cope with unexpected delays and emergencies.

The foregoing should enable one to appreciate why it is necessary to enquire fully into all food and drink consumed during the 24 hours immediately prior to a criminal incident. It may provide the additional evidence required to clinch the diagnosis.

❑ Education

For the woman it could be a tremendous relief, or it may come as a shock, to realise that she suffers from severe premenstrual syndrome. The unexplainable, but ever present mood changes, may have been there for many years and the blame first placed on other factors or it was assumed to be part of her normal personality. It is important that each woman understands her own problem, learns to recognise her earliest warning symptoms and knows how to react to prevent catastrophes occurring. She must fully understand her personal medication and the importance of the dietary regime. All women are different and have individual needs in treatment and education.

Severe sufferers must be taught to resist being lured by advertised medicaments of dubious value or brainwashed into believing that over-the-counter remedies will solve their hormonal problems. It has been widely suggested that deficiencies of vitamins or trace minerals are the cause of premenstrual syndrome, but why should deficiencies of these vitamins and minerals cause premenstrual syndrome in women and not in men? In women only just before menstruation and not after menstruation? In women before menstruation and not when they are pregnant and nourishing a growing fetus? – And why in some women and not in all women? There is no evidence of true deficiencies of vitamins or minerals amongst the people of Britain.

Sufferers of premenstrual syndrome should especially avoid vitamin B6, or pyridoxine, which is not needed in the western world where no cases of vitamin B6 deficiency occur, but also because it can cause nerve damage or peripheral neuritis when used even in small doses and intermittently. Research workers trying out drugs for the treatment of peripheral neuritis use vitamin B6 to induce peripheral neuritis in the laboratory animals they are using for their tests. So why give it to humans? Studies of women have shown that when blood levels of vitamin B6 are above average neurological signs develop after six months in some 60% of women taking B6 (Dalton and Dalton 1987). Initially it causes pins and needles in the hands and feet, areas of numbness, hypersensitivity of the skin and muscle weakness so that the hand grip is too poor to open bottles, they have difficulty in running and climbing stairs, and ultimately they may become wheelchair bound if their dosage of vitamin B6 was grossly excessive such as occurred in Americans reported by Schaumberg *et al* 1983.

Night work is deleterious to sufferers of premenstrual syndrome. The centre for the control of day/night rhythm is situated in the hypothalamus at the base of the brain adjacent to the menstrual regulating centre and if disturbed may cause an increase in severity of premenstrual syndrome. It is particularly tempting for nurses, after they have had a child, to offer to do night work once or twice a week. The husband can care for the child overnight, the extra cash is useful and it keeps her skills up to date, but she pays a price in sleep disturbance. Similarly women with premenstrual syndrome need to be warned that they are prone to suffer from jet lag, and must ensure if travelling on business to have adequate recovery time on landing.

Discussion and advice is needed on contraception, as all oral contraceptives contain progestogens which lower blood progesterone level and so increase premenstrual symptoms. The advice must be to stop the pill and find some other method of contraception. Sterilization, also, increases the severity of premenstrual syndrome and should be avoided, and reversal of tubal sterilization will not improve premenstrual syndrome. However, progesterone can be used as a reliable contraceptive method for severe sufferers of premenstrual syndrome (Dalton *et al* 1987). Women planning a pregnancy should be advised to consider having progesterone prophylaxis for the prevention of postnatal depression, in which case the progesterone is started at the completion of labour and given in decreasing doses until the return of menstruation (Dalton 1985 and 1989).

> A 21 years old secretary was seen the day after she had tried to strangle her boy friend, and when she had just started menstruation. On the previous month she had taken an overdose on the immediate premenstrual day and been admitted to the Royal Infirmary. She had made 28 previous threats of suicide, apparently always in the premenstruum, so she had been referred to the gynaecologist, who prescribed vitamin B6 50 mg daily. A full consultation revealed that she was on the pill, and that she normally avoided all forms of starchy food, as well as having no food whatsoever between breakfast and an evening meal. She was advised to stop the pill and vitamin B6 immediately, and instructed about the need for three hourly starchy snacks. The dietary advice and education was probably more important in her case than the progesterone therapy, which she was also given.

Women, whose premenstrual syndrome is so severe that the possibility exists that they might be brought before the courts, should not be considered for double blind controlled trials of drugs, as these demand a couple of months observation without any treatment, followed by a further month or two on placebo during which time there could be several recurrences of symptoms with the danger of criminal involvement.

❑ References

Dalton K (1984). *Premenstrual Syndrome and Progesterone Therapy;* 2nd Ed. William Heinemann Medical Books Ltd/Year Book Medical Publications Inc Chicago.

Dalton K. (1985). *Practitioner;* **229**, 507-508.

Dalton K. (1989). *J. Psychosomat Obstet & Gynaec;* **10**, Supp 1, 143.

Dalton M.E., Guthrie K. & Dalton K. (1987). *Brit J. Family Planning;* **13**, 87-89.

Dalton K. & Dalton M.J.T. (1987). *Acta Neuro Scand;* **76**, 8-11.

Greene R & Dalton K (1953). *Brit Med J.;* **1**, 1007.

Schaumberg *et al* (1983). *N. Engl J. Med;* 309, 445-447.

14

Failure to Recognise

Woman's behaviour problems have been known for thousands of years, but most of the knowledge, understanding and scientific interest has come in only the last forty years since a successful treatment for premenstrual syndrome has been found and used. Only in the last five years has the aetiology begun to unfold. Even so, it is barely the tip of the iceberg that has come into view. The failure of the medical profession to recognise the progress that has been made is matched by the failure to recognise and bring relief to those severe sufferers whose lives are being blighted with criminal stigma for acts of which they have no recollection whatsoever or may only vaguely realise that something occurred. These acts were performed under the influence of irresistible impulses engendered by their premenstrual syndrome.

In the various chapters of this book readers will have learned of the consequences of that failure of recognition, but it is difficult to convey in words what nightmares, sufferings and damages are perpetuated by that failure. Those who have been treated unjustly and in whom the problems of premenstrual syndrome were not recognised early enough, tend to bear a grudge against society. They themselves cannot explain their bizarre behaviour, only knowing that something is wrong, but they don't understand why, what or wherefore. No one will listen to their crazy stories of their hallucinations or delusions compelling some unusual action against their will. They are judged by logical minds who do not and cannot understand the total illogicality of their confused minds. Often they are in a dazed state, some even sleep it off, and are then accused of an action they cannot recall doing. They wake up to a nightmare that is really true. The evidence is there, the witnesses are ready to testify. They were seen to fight, stab, behave violently or steal. They must have done it, although they have no recollection of the act. When at last they receive the reassurance of a diagnosis and find the relief that comes with treatment, they cannot really be blamed for feeling resentful, reproaching the world and welfare state for that failure to recognise that it all happened because the body's chemicals went awry.

Too often the answer is found too late, after years of misunderstanding, incredible mistakes, broken friendships, disrupted marriages, parental estrangement and the stigma of criminality. The sudden antisocial behaviour of a pubertal girl has a disruptive influence on her family, most have no previous family history of conflict with the law. Parents are out of their depth, unable to understand and with no knowledge of how to deal with the situation. In their shame they are frightened to discuss the problem with those who might be able to help, their doctor, social worker, probation officer, teacher or religious advisor. Parent's inability to deal with the daughter brings new pressures on them, which serve either to bring them closer together or force them further apart, ultimately separating and leaving their unfortunate daughter without the help and support she truly needs at this vital time.

If the worst happens and this sick girl is imprisoned or sent for corrective detention, she will meet a totally different type of offender, one who has known conflict with the law since early childhood, whose parents know their rights, all the dodges and how to avoid detection. She will unconsciously learn more about crime, wilful crime, crime and its handsome rewards, crime with a worthwhile motive and the many tricks to avoid detection and supply alibis. In this closed community, new friendships are formed from shared experiences which continue in the outside world where harassment and rejection await.

In prison there is loss of personal responsibility. No longer is there a need to worry about money, buying and cooking food, living arrangements or the daily chore of school or finding employment. It is institutionalisation at its worst. The result is that emotional maturity is halted during the years of imprisonment and on being discharged the offender comes out at the same stage of development as she went in. Meanwhile the other seventeen year olds they knew before going to prison have matured emotionally and physically and are now self-supporting, and having had their brief love affairs they have now decided what they want from life and the general direction of their future. Not so for the offender, who is now emotionally younger than her chronological age. Her life is tough with no work, for who wants to employ her when there is a wide selection of others to choose from? Who needs the friendship of an immature girl of doubtful background, harassed by neighbours and pointed out by the boys? Her need is the restoration of confidence, trust and friendship, but in practice this is difficult to achieve.

One offender mentioned that another girl she had met in prison while they were both receiving progesterone treatment was still unemployed. 'Jean must learn to lie – it's the only way out – she must live the lie – be able to explain her absence by a trip to some far away town and know all about the town'. But I knew Jean better, she was too honest to concoct a lie, even if it was for her personal benefit.

The PMS Action Inc. of Wisconsin introduced the parents of two premenstrual syndrome teenagers living a thousand miles apart. When the girls met they spent a whole day in a room recalling together their similar experiences, with alternating laughter and tears. Only they knew what it was like to wake up and not be believed, with no one understanding and completely unable to offer a reasonable explanation for their absurd behaviour. Meanwhile, next door, the parents discussed the changes which had come over their daughters as they moved into puberty, and the difficulty they had, once having made the connection between the days of disturbed behaviour and menstruation, in finding anyone who would believe them, much less offer treatment or any hope. Both had, in fact, ended up by asking for help in a transatlantic 'phone call.

But offenders are not limited to those whose problems started at puberty. In the older age groups are those whose problems arose with the pill, after a pregnancy particularly if followed by postnatal depression, or after their family was complete and the decision was made to have a sterilisation. These mature women do not experience the halting of emotional development, but for them the sudden mood swings are just as difficult to comprehend. Having reached maturity as law abiding citizens, married with a family and maintaining the same ideals and morals of earlier years, it is most disturbing to discover they are no longer in full control of their tempers or alcoholic urges. They have brought up their children to respect the law only to find that they themselves transgress against their will and beyond their control.

Initially the mature woman tries to keep the problem to herself. Many are the confidences heard of how an honest woman tries to return her stolen goods. She didn't want them, dare not tell her husband and is frightened her children will find out. It would seem that it is much easier to take items from shops when in a daze than it is to return them when clear minded.

Premenstrual syndrome ranks among the diseases in which the sympathy and understanding of the husband can be of greatest value. First he must understand the reason for the period changes in his wife's personality over which neither she nor he has any control. She would like to be calm, happy and loving every day, not just for half the month, but her chemical imbalance denies her this. Without the understanding husband the marriage breaks, for who wants to live forever with a volcanic wife about to erupt unexpectedly at any time?

In France at a medical meeting on premenstrual syndrome, the cyclical occurrences of violence, as revealed by the prison documents, was being discussed. A woman prison medical officer recalled just such a case under her care. The files had confirmed the episodes of misbehaviour were related to menstruation; however, she did not help the woman, nor use her findings in evidence for her defence as, 'the climate of medical knowledge in France was not yet ready for such a defence as premenstrual syndrome'. The other discussants were forceful in reminding her that her duty was to help the prisoner, without regard to public opinion or fear of media pressure. She was a doctor to whom the prisoner had come for help; it was her duty to provide the best possible treatment and advice.

Once the disease is recognised and treatment instituted, there lies ahead the task of trying to mend the marriage, restart old friendships, and progress in one's employment. There is no future in looking back in anger or with resentment at the failure to recognise the plight earlier.

> An unknown woman wrote, 'Thank you, your treatment has got me back to normal, and saved a marriage which was on the rocks and would otherwise have ended in

divorce, like that of so many other PMS sufferers. Let's hope the doctors sit up and recognise this time of the month and treat it. You have started a mighty big ball rolling. I hope it gets up steam'.

There can be no question about it. The failure to recognise and treat premenstrual syndrome is tragic for some women, but failure to recognise premenstrual syndrome as a mitigating factor in criminal behaviour can be utterly disastrous.

15

Jumping on the Bandwagon

It remains to emphasise that the premenstrual syndrome, which has been so rigidly defined and diagnosed, is not an easy option for mitigation. It should also be viewed as a difficult option, especially as it entails a promise to accept treatment to ensure the offence does not recur. The very purpose of the rigid definition, which has been repeatedly stressed in this book, is to prevent the malingerer and her legal advisers from jumping on the bandwagon and falsely claiming premenstrual syndrome where it does not exist. Admittedly, one lawyer confided to me that his first duty is to his client and whilst there are still many on the judiciary who do not know or understand premenstrual syndrome, it is only right that he should try and plead premenstrual syndrome in mitigation in all possible cases. However, while it is not possible to stop the lawyer from trying, if his attempt is unfounded, it does not help the real sufferer nor does it further the course of justice.

> A 'phone call from a general practitioner in Colchester, Essex, expressed his annoyance that the jury had neglected to consider or recognise his diagnosis of premenstrual syndrome in a shoplifting charge against one of his patients. The doctor admitted that it was her first offence, there had been no record of menstruation although the offence had occurred 'near the time of menstruation', there had been no previous premenstrual symptoms, there were no notes of her having suffered from premenstrual syndrome in his medical records and she had never received treatment for it. No witnesses were called. The doctor and perhaps the woman's lawyer had naively hoped that the mere statement that the woman suffered from premenstrual syndrome would be accepted without further ado.

Barbara Newman, assistant district attorney for New York State, claimed before the Food and Drug Administration in

February 1983 in Washington that, 'because of difficulties diagnosing premenstrual syndrome it can be easily feigned and just as easily attributed to women who do not have it'... and later... 'Given the difficulty of proving or disproving the presence or absence of premenstrual syndrome, a woman would have a hard time disproving the allegation'. (Newman 1983). On the contrary, in Britain at least it is difficult to produce false evidence of pre-eclampsia, postnatal depression, termination of pregnancy, or sterilisation as all these medical events are recorded in the medical notes held by the general practitioner. Professor Michael Drury, (1983) head of general practice at Birmingham, wisely reminded general practitioners of the importance of entering premenstrual syndrome in their medical records, as the importance of a plea of mitigation is almost in inverse ratio to its non importance as a defence of premenstrual syndrome.

> On 16th December, 1981, a 24 year American mother of six children was arrested on her first criminal charge of assaulting her four year daughter with her hand or a stick, causing soft tissue injury to the girl's waist and knees. *Initially* she pleaded premenstrual syndrome, and it was to be the first time that the defence was to be used in the States. Although the act occurred in the premenstruum she had no record of menstruation, her six pregnancies had all been normal with no complications of threatened abortion, pre-eclampsia or postnatal depression, and she reported no side effects on the pill although she had since been sterilised. Her diagnostic checklist score was low at 22% and her SHBG estimation was within normal levels. Furthermore she was not receiving nor did she intend to receive treatment for her alleged premenstrual syndrome.

In effect she was asking the judge to return her six children to her care so that she could continue to abuse them every premenstruum. She did not suffer from premenstrual syndrome and her plea was wisely withdrawn. Instead, she pleaded guilty and used harassment as a mitigating factor. Had Ms. Newman been defending this American woman in a plea of premenstrual syndrome instead of prosecuting she would have had a hard task indeed.

Mention has already been made that the mere fact, that an alleged offence occurred in the premenstruum is not evidence of premenstrual syndrome. Such occurrences could have been a coincidence. Further evidence is required (Chapter 11).

One applauds the move by the larger stores to prosecute all shoplifters and leave it to the courts to differentiate the wrong-doers from the sick women. The move is a necessary precaution as large sums are lost annually from shop thefts. It is the law abiding citizen who suffers, as the loss is inevitably passed on to the customer in the form of higher charges. It has proved effective, for instance, in stopping the flow of individuals who visit Oxford Street, London, with only one purpose, that of shoplifting. The habitual shoplifters are easily spotted by the store detectives, because they are often acting in pairs, possibly a woman and child, and maybe wearing a coat with poacher's pockets. The number of cases of shoplifting in which premenstrual syndrome is genuinely a factor is infinitesimal. If a court appearance leads to its diagnosis and ultimate treatment nothing but good will result. One must not let every shoplifter jump on the bandwagon.

> A 25 year old unemployed woman was charged with attempted murder and the plea of premenstrual syndrome was suggested as a cause of diminished responsibility. During her medical examination in prison she requested a hysterectomy, as menstruation was so heavy, and the removal of her breasts, so that she could go out into the world as a man. Although she did have serious problems of sexual identity, there was no evidence of premenstrual syndrome.

Following a talk to the Association of Police Surgeons of Great Britain on 'Criminal Violence and Premenstrual Syndrome' *The Times* stated on the front page 'The Pill and Sterilisation cause Crime'. The result of *'The Times'* report of the talk was, that several teenagers were referred for investigation into the possibility of their suffering from premenstrual syndrome. They all had a history of violence and were in different detention centres in Britain. Although their problems had all started at puberty, they were not all suffering from premenstrual syndrome. However, on full examination some girls were noted to have excess hair of the masculine type, and their blood tests showed high levels of testosterone and dihydrotestosterone, the male hormones (Dalton 1981). These girls all had psychiatric reports before they had been sent to the detention centres, but not necessarily full examinations. They had removed their facial hair with electrolysis or wax, they were wearing long sleeves and jeans so the other excess hair would not be spotted unless they were seen undressed. There is a happy ending to their story in that although some did not have premenstrual syndrome, those with raised testosterone levels started on treatment with a special anti-testosterone drug, called cyproterone acetate, which lowers testosterone levels. These girls lost their excessive hair and also their violent tempers. Four at least have now graduated from colleges of further education, and all are useful law abiding citizens.

Sometimes a 'bandwagon' can lead to a greater understanding of a problem, but only if all who are involved make themselves fully conversant with what is true and what is false. As to whether the use of the premenstrual syndrome as a factor of mitigation becomes a 'bandwagon', depends on sufficient numbers of the legal and medical professions being prepared to become fully informed and their determination to ensure that it does not become one.

❑ References

Dalton K. (1981). *Neuropharmacology;* **20**, 1267-1269.
Drury M. (1983). *Pulse;* May 8th.
Newman B. (1983). *Evidence Public Enquiry into Progesterone for Premenstrual Syndrome;* Washington. Feb.

16

Conclusion

The information contained in this book is firmly based on the factual clinical experience of the author and not on armchair theorising. That clinical experience with premenstrual syndrome began in 1948 and has continued unabated to this day. It would be quite incorrect to imply that women's untreated premenstrual syndrome will inevitably end up in the criminal courts. Unfortunately some small numbers of women do, but such cases form only a very small proportion of those suffering from premenstrual syndrome. Theirs is an extremely severe form, which is a very rare but very real condition. Nevertheless, it responds just as completely to the correct treatment with progesterone as do all other forms of the disease.

Physicians and psychiatrists have been trained to make diagnoses from observations of symptoms and signs and from the results of investigations. With premenstrual syndrome, however, the diagnosis depends on a specific time relationship in the menstrual cycle. Psychiatrists and psychologists have studied premenstrual syndrome from their special viewpoint and found no specific symptoms to differentiate premenstrual syndrome from other psychiatric disorders. It is only when viewed from a gynaecological endocrinological standpoint, looking at timing of events and not at symptoms, that other hormonal correlates emerge to assist in the diagnosis. For instance, the time of onset and of increased severity of the disease is at times of hormonal crisis. There is an inability to tolerate oral contraceptives, a high incidence of pre-eclampsia and also of postnatal depression or there is the finding of a low sex hormone binding globulin binding capacity (SHBG). All these factors have pointed to a hormonal diagnosis and the need for the strict definition.

The realisation that some cases of very severe premenstrual syndrome can be responsible for criminal acts can also mean that any criminal act which does not appear to have any logical motive, or is a recurrent offence, should always be referred for investigations to exclude the possibility of premenstrual syndrome for which help is available. Treatment will not only restore the woman to society as a law abiding person but it will also make economic sense. The cost of treatment with progesterone (based on an average dose) would be £14 for one month's treatment with suppositories or £5 with injections. The cost of keeping her in prison for one month would be £700, so for the cost of keeping one woman in prison 50 of the premenstrual syndrome offenders could be safe, well and free (Figure 16.1).

The essential knowledge required, by all who are concerned with those sufferers from premenstrual syndrome whose behaviour brings them into conflict with the law, is to be found in the foregoing chapters. This does not mean that this volume contains all that is known about this disease. That would require a much larger book. The somatic presentations have not been touched upon, and are to be found in the book for the medical profession (Dalton 1984). Research is going on in

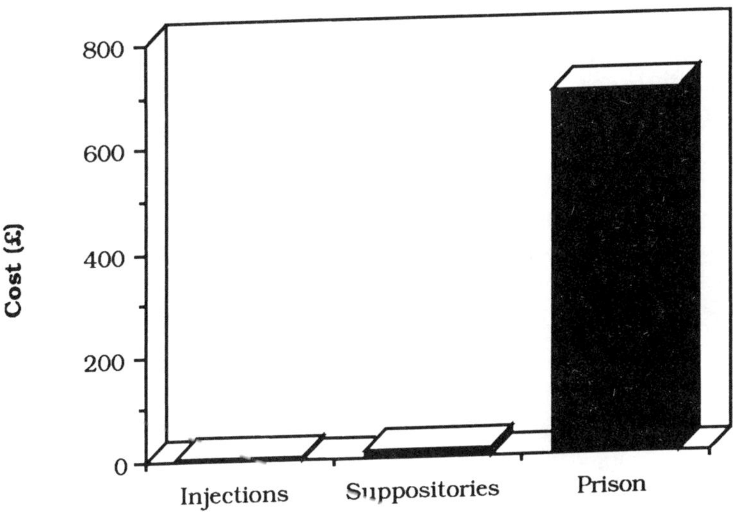

Figure 16.1 Comparative costs of one month's treatment and one month's imprisonment.

many scientific disciplines and adding to our knowledge almost daily. If the benefits of such work are to be utilised much work has to be done in the education of all those involved. Special courses of training will be needed for prison officers, teachers, lawyers, police, health visitors, social workers, and general practitioners . All should be made aware of the need for early recognition and treatment before the calamity occurs .

If premenstrual syndrome is to continue being used as a plea of diminished responsibility or mitigation, there must be a strict adherence to the definition and diagnosis as set down in the earlier chapters, and a demonstration, for the protection of the public, that there has been a complete response to progesterone treatment before the woman is returned into society, where the responsibility for monitoring her progress will rest with her general practitioner and the health visitor. These necessary facilities are available in this country and are being used. It is a different story, however, in the United States for, although there is great interest in the legal implication, there is a scarcity of correct information. Progesterone is not yet universally available, nor have progesterone suppositories been recognised as efficacious by the Food and Drug Administration.

In the end it is the duty of society to ensure that the genuine sufferer of premenstrual syndrome receives treatment and not a criminal record, whilst at the same time ensuring that the malingerer does not benefit from a false plea.

❑ Reference

Dalton K. (1984). *Premenstrual Syndrome and Progesterone Therapy;* William Heinemann Med. Books Ltd. London/Year Book Medical Publishers Inc. Chicago. 2nd Edition.

Glossary

Actus reus – the guilty act.
Aetiology – cause of disease.
Adrenalin – one of many hormones produced by the adrenal glands.
Amnesia – loss of memory.
Analgesics – pain relievers.
Anorexia – loss of appetite.
Anovular – without ovulation.
Atrophy – diminution of size and functional activity.
Diuretics – drugs which increase the output of urine.
Dysmenorrhoea– a pain with menstruation.
Endometrium – inner lining of the womb.
Fallopian tubes – two tubes leading from the ovaries to the womb along which the egg cells pass.
Follicular phase – days from menstruation to ovulation.
Follicle Stimulating Hormone (FSH) – hormone from pituitary which acts on the ovary stimulating oestrogen production and maturation of the ovum.
Glaucoma – disease of the eye characterised by raised pressure in the eye.
Gonadotrophins – hormones stimulating production of sex hormones, i. e. FSH and LH.
Homicide – the act of killing another person.
Hormones – chemical messengers produced by glands, which pass into the blood stream to exert an action at a distant site.
Hormone receptors – transporters of hormone molecules through the cell wall to the nucleus.
Hyperglycaemia – rise in blood sugar level above the normal.
Hypertrophy – increase in size.
Hypoglycaemia – reduction of blood sugar level below the normal.
Hypothalamus – specialised area of the hind brain concerned with controlling mechanisms, including menstruation.
Hysterectomy – removal of the womb.

Implant – pellets of drugs inserted into the tissue for prolonged action

Insane – of unsound mind, mentally deranged.

Intermenstruum – part of the menstrual cycle not covered by premenstruum or menstruation.

Libido – sexual urge.

Luteal phase – days from ovulation to menstruation.

Luteinising Hormone (LH) – hormone from pituitary which acts on the ovary stimulating ovulation and the production of progesterone.

Manslaughter – criminal homicide without malice aforethought.

Menarche – the first menstruation.

Menopause – last menstruation marking the end of childbearing.

Mens rea – the guilty intent.

Menstrual cycle – time from first day of menstruation to the first day of next menstruation.

Menstrual distress – symptoms throughout the menstrual cycle which become worse during the paramenstruum.

Menstrual flow – blood lost at menstruation.

Menstruation – monthly bleeding from the vagina in women of childbearing age, caused by the disintegration of the lining of the womb.

Metabolism – building up and breaking down of chemicals in the body.

Migraine – severe form of headache.

Mitigation – lessening the severity.

Nymphomania – excessive sexual urges.

Oedema – accumulation of fluid in the tissues.

Oestrogen – hormone produced by the ovaries which produces female characteristics.

Oophorectomy – removal of one or both ovaries.

Ovulation – release of egg cell from the ovary.

Ovum – egg cell.

Paramenstruum – four days before menstruation and the first four days of menstruation.

Paranoia – mental disease with delusions of persecution.

Pituitary gland – situated immediately below the brain which manufactures numerous hormones.

Placebo – inactive drug given in clinical trials.
Placenta – organ produced in the womb during pregnancy to nourish the foetus, which is connected to the placenta by the umbilical cord.
Polysymptomatic – having numerous different symptoms.
Postmenstruum – days immediately after menstruation.
Postnatal – after childbirth.
Preeclampsia or preeclamptic toxaemia – disease of pregnancy characterised by high blood pressure, oedema and protein in urine.
Premenstruum – days immediately before menstruation.
Progesterone – hormone produced by the ovary after ovulation, by the placenta in pregnancy, and by the adrenal where it is immediately converted into numerous corticosteroids.
Progestogens – synthetic drugs used in contraception, once thought to be true progesterone substitutes.
Prophylactic – preventative.
Psychosis – mental derangement not due to neurosis or depression.
Puberty – the age at which a child becomes capable of procreation.
Puerperal – after childbirth (adj).
Puerperium – days after child birth.
Sex hormone binding globulin – a minute protein to which the sex hormones bind as they are transported in the blood.
Symptom – a complaint by a patient of an abnormal condition.
Synchrony – at the same time.
Syndrome – collection of symptoms which commonly occur together.
Tanycytes – brain cells which pass information about the composition of the cerebrospinal fluid to the hypothalamus.
Testosterone – hormone which produces masculine characteristics.
Therapy – treatment.
Thyroxine – hormone produced by the thyroid gland.
Uterus – womb.
Vagina – passage leading from exterior of body to the womb.
Vertigo – giddiness.

Further Reading by the Author

'Once a Month', 1987. 4th Edition, Fontana/Collins, London, and Hunter House, Pomona, California. 5th Edition USA 1990: UK 1991.

'Depression after Childbirth', 1989, 2nd Edition, Oxford University Press, Oxford.

'Premenstrual Syndrome and Progesterone Therapy', 1984, 2nd Edition, William Heinemann Medical Books, London.

'Effect of Menstruation on Schoolgirls' Weekly Work', 1960, British Medical Journal, 2, 1425.

'Schoolgirls' Behaviour and Menstruation', 1960, British Medical Journal, 2, 1649.

'Menstruation and Crime', 1961, British Medical Journal, 2, 1752.

'Menstruation and Examinations', 1968, Lancet, ii, 1386.

'Cyclical Criminal Acts in Premenstrual Syndrome', 1980, Lancet, 1070-1071.

'The Legal Implications of Premenstrual Syndrome', 1982, World Medicine, 17th April.

'Behaviour and the Menstrual Cycle', (1982) Ed: Friedman R.C., Marcel Dekker Inc., New York & Basle: K. Dalton, Chap: 11.

'Premenstrual Syndrome: A New Criminal Defence, 1982, Laurence Taylor and K. Dalton, Californian Western Law Review.

'Legal Implications of PMS', 1986, Hamline Law Review, 9, 1, 143-154.

'Premenstrual Syndrome – Ethical and Legal Implications – a Biomedical Perspective', 1987, Ed: Ginsburg B.E. & Carter B.F., Plenum Press, New York & London, 287-300.

Index